LIVING FIT & STRONG

Vol. 2

Simple Chair Exercises To Lose Weight, Regain Independence And Mobility For Seniors Over 70

DR. THOMPSON CLARK

TABLE OF CONTENTS

ABOUT THE AUTHOR

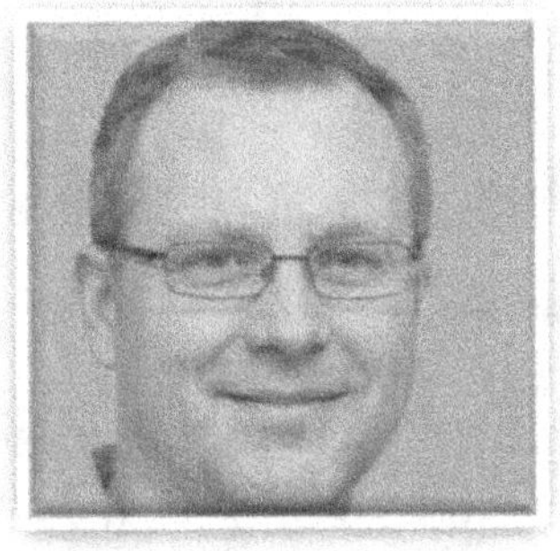 **Dr. Thompson Clark** is a seasoned physical therapist and geriatric care specialist with over 30 years of experience working to improve the lives of older individuals. Dr. Clark, a specialist in mobility, flexibility, and pain treatment, has established himself as a respected figure in senior health, advocating for non-invasive approaches that assist older people in preserving their freedom. His desire to help seniors stay active and healthy has led him to create simple stretching routines adapted to their specific needs.

Dr. Clark's schooling includes a *Doctorate of Physical Therapy (DPT)* with a focus on geriatric care. Early in his work, he noticed a void in elder healthcare: exercise and mobility were frequently disregarded in favor of medication or surgery. In response, he developed individualized programs to manage chronic pain, flexibility, and posture, allowing elders to enjoy pain-free, satisfying lives. His method emphasizes the importance of simple, effective exercises that anyone can undertake, regardless of fitness level.

As an author, Dr. Clark has written extensively about senior health and wellness, making complicated medical concepts simple for his readers. His books and articles highlight the benefits of stretching and movement for older people, providing practical recommendations that seniors can adopt into their everyday routines. His writing has a devoted audience due to his ability to explain health information without compromising depth or accuracy.

In addition to his professional practice and writing, Dr. Clark is a prominent advocate for seniors' mental and emotional well-being. He incorporates mindfulness and relaxation techniques into his stretching sessions, which assist older folks manage stress and anxiety while improving their physical health. His holistic approach emphasizes the link between mind and body, encouraging elders to look after both parts of their well-being.

Dr. Clark is active in his community, providing free workshops and wellness initiatives for seniors, particularly in impoverished regions. His dedication to keeping older individuals active and healthy extends beyond his professional career, as he continues to educate healthcare workers and promote wellness programs that enable seniors to live their best lives.

INTRODUCTION

Maintaining physical health becomes more vital as we become older, but it is also more difficult. For seniors over 70, staying active is about more than simply bodily health; it's about maintaining independence, improving quality of life, and increasing overall well-being. Unfortunately, standard exercise routines can be challenging for older persons due to joint pain, mobility limitations, or fear of damage. This is where chair exercises come in.

Chair exercises are a safe, effective, and easily accessible alternative for elders to remain physically active. They provide a gentler form of movement that supports the body while reducing joint strain, making them excellent for persons who have difficulty standing for lengthy periods or moving freely. Chair exercises may be performed practically anywhere—at home, at a community center, or even in a wheelchair—allowing seniors to keep active without needing costly gym subscriptions or fancy equipment.

This book is intended to guide elders through exercises aimed at boosting strength, flexibility, balance, and cardiovascular health. The exercises provided in this book can help you reach your goals of losing weight, regaining lost mobility, or simply staying active and independent.

Many seniors confront challenges that make standard exercise programs impossible. Conditions including arthritis, osteoporosis, balance challenges, and chronic pain can make it difficult to participate in high-impact or vigorous sports. Furthermore, fear of falling or injury can cause some older persons to forego exercising entirely, even though staying active is one of the most important things they can do for their health.

Many of these restrictions are eliminated with chair exercises. They allow elders to remain sitting while performing exercises that improve flexibility, strength, and cardiovascular health. The chair provides support for the body, reducing the risk of damage from falls or overexertion. Chair exercises are also very adjustable, which means they may be tailored to individuals with varied fitness levels and physical abilities. This makes them ideal for seniors who are just starting a fitness regimen or those recovering from an injury or sickness.

Another significant advantage of chair exercises is that they promote consistency. They can be done from the comfort of your own home, eliminating the need for transportation or access to a gym. This adaptability makes it easier to include regular exercise into your daily routine, which is essential for long-term health and wellness.

This book is structured into chapters that walk readers through the various facets of chair exercises, giving a comprehensive approach to fitness. The chapters are meant to help you start cautiously and grow at your own pace, with emphasis on various aspects of health such as strength, flexibility, balance, and heart health.

Starting an exercise regimen might be scary, especially if you've been sedentary for a long. However, with chair exercises, you are taking the first step toward a healthier, more active lifestyle—one in which you can restore strength, mobility, and independence.

This book is intended to help you along your path by providing simple workouts and practical recommendations customized to your specific needs. Regardless of your current fitness level, chair workouts are a safe and effective method to keep active, lose weight, and enhance your quality of life.

Incorporating chair workouts into your daily routine not only improves your physical health but also invests in your future. You're gaining control over your body and your well-being, allowing you to focus on the activities and experiences that are most important.

Now, let's get started on the path to fitness and strength.

CHAPTER 1: UNDERSTANDING THE FUNDAMENTALS OF CHAIR EXERCISES

Definition And Benefits Of Chair Exercises

Chair exercises are a type of physical activity that is conducted while seated in a chair, offering a low-impact, accessible workout option for people with restricted mobility, particularly seniors. These exercises can target a variety of fitness goals, including strength, flexibility, balance, and cardiovascular health, without needing participants to stand or carry their entire body weight. These exercises, which use the support of a chair, provide a safe and effective approach to maintaining or enhancing physical fitness, particularly for individuals recuperating from accidents, managing chronic conditions, or looking for gentle ways to keep active.

Chair exercises typically consist of seated movements like arm lifts, leg extensions, and torso twists. To provide stability during standing exercises, they may use resistance bands, light weights, or the back of a chair. Despite their simplicity, chair exercises may provide a full-body workout and can be tailored to a range of fitness levels, from beginner to experienced. Chair exercises can be tailored to individual needs, making them a versatile fitness alternative for weight loss, flexibility improvement, and strength development.

While chair exercises have several health benefits, their advantages over other types of exercise make them ideal for the elderly or individuals with physical limitations. *Here's an explanation of why chair workouts stand out and provide distinct benefits:*

1. Suitable for all Fitness Levels

One of the most notable benefits of chair exercises is that they are accessible to people of all fitness levels, particularly those who struggle with standing or high-impact activities. Traditional types of exercise, such as jogging, jumping, or lifting weights, can be difficult for those who have mobility limitations, joint problems, or chronic illnesses like arthritis. Chair exercises, on the other hand, provide a supportive environment in which motions are carried out while seated, greatly lowering strain on joints, bones, and muscles.

For beginners or those returning to fitness after a lengthy absence, chair exercises provide an entry point into physical activity without the risk of injury or overexertion. They allow people to gain confidence and progressively increase their fitness without having to conduct more difficult or demanding workouts.

2. Safety and Lower Risk of Injury

Many seniors and others with health concerns prioritize safety, and chair workouts provide a significant advantage in this regard. Exercises performed from a seated position reduce the chance of losing balance or falling, which is especially beneficial for persons with limited coordination or weak muscles. This is critical because falls are one of the main causes of injury among older persons, frequently resulting in fractures or other severe problems.

Furthermore, the supporting structure of a chair reduces the pressure on joints and bones, making these workouts easier on the body. Chair exercises allow persons with arthritis or osteoporosis to keep active without causing pain or discomfort. The controlled movements also decrease the possibility of overextending muscles or tendons, making chair exercises a safe option for people with previous injuries or medical issues.

3. Adaptability to Individual Needs

One of the most intriguing aspects of chair workouts is their versatility. These workouts are simply adaptable to match the demands of various individuals. Chair exercises can be altered in intensity and complexity to suit a complete beginner, someone recovering from surgery, or anyone looking for a more challenging workout.

Resistance bands or light hand weights, for example, can be used to make certain movements more challenging, while people who want more assistance can adhere to simple, moderate exercises. In this approach, chair workouts can address a wide range of fitness objectives, from strength development to flexibility enhancement, all within the same framework.

Chair exercises can also be customized to target certain regions of the body, such as the legs, arms, or core. This makes them especially handy for people who want to concentrate on a certain location without straining other sections of their bodies. For example, someone recovering from knee surgery can focus on upper body strength without having to stand or put pressure on their lower body.

4. Convenience and Little Equipment Requirements

Another advantage of chair exercises is that they are convenient. They can be done practically any place, as long as a stable chair is present. There is no requirement for a gym membership or specialized equipment, making them an appealing option for people who may struggle to access traditional training facilities.

Chair exercises are perfect for seniors who like to exercise at home. All you need is a sturdy chair, and alternative equipment such as light weights or resistance bands can be added for variation, but they are not required. This makes chair exercises inexpensive and straightforward to include in a regular program, regardless of the individual's living arrangements.

Chair exercises are also portable, allowing them to be performed in tiny locations, which is useful for people who live in apartments, assisted living facilities, or smaller homes. Because of the minimum space and equipment needs, seniors and people with restricted mobility can remain active without the logistical issues associated with bigger training sets.

5. Integration with Daily Life

Chair workouts have the distinct advantage of being easily incorporated into everyday life. Unlike more sophisticated workout regimens, which may necessitate devoted time and focus, chair exercises can frequently be completed in small spurts throughout the day. This ability to split exercise into smaller periods can help elders and people with busy schedules be consistent with physical activity.

A person could, for example, do a series of leg lifts while watching television or stretch their upper body while seated at a desk or dining table. This flexibility makes it easier to keep to a regimen because there is no need to set out a significant amount of time for exercise. Instead, chair workouts can be incorporated into regular activities, making them a long-term fitness solution.

6. Low-impact, yet Effective

While chair exercises are low-impact and mild on the joints, they can nevertheless be quite helpful in improving strength, flexibility, and cardiovascular fitness. Many people believe that a seated workout cannot be as intense as standing exercises; nevertheless, with the proper movements and changes, chair exercises can give a hard and full workout.

Upper body activities, such as sitting bicep curls or seated chest presses, can efficiently enhance muscle strength, whilst seated marches or toe taps can increase heart rate for a cardiovascular workout. Chair exercises are controlled and allow for targeted muscle engagement, so individuals can still grow muscle and improve fitness without standing or executing high-intensity motions.

7. Suitable for Rehabilitation and Chronic Conditions

Another significant benefit of chair workouts is their applicability to people undergoing rehabilitation or treating chronic health conditions. Traditional exercise programs frequently put too much strain on recuperating muscles, bones, or joints, slowing recovery or exacerbating symptoms of specific illnesses. Chair exercises, on the other hand, are soft enough to be included in a rehabilitation program for persons recovering from operations, accidents, or diseases.

Individuals with chronic diseases such as arthritis, osteoporosis, or cardiovascular disease benefit from chair exercises since they are low-impact and promote movement, which is crucial for overall health. Regular movement can help to alleviate stiffness, promote blood flow, and prevent muscle weakness, all of which are important for managing chronic diseases. Chair exercises, in particular, serve to avoid the loss of mobility that can occur after prolonged periods of inactivity by providing a safe and effective technique to keep the body moving.

Physical therapists frequently add chair exercises into rehabilitation plans because they help patients develop strength, flexibility, and range of motion without putting undue strain on sensitive areas. For example, someone recovering from hip or knee surgery can work on strengthening their upper body or core while seated, gradually improving their overall fitness and preparing their body to return to more traditional types of exercise.

8. Supports independence and aging in place

Many older persons prioritize maintaining their independence, and chair exercises can help elders stay self-sufficient for extended periods. People's muscle strength, balance, and flexibility may deteriorate as they age, making common actions like getting out of bed, rising from a chair, or walking short distances more difficult. Chair exercises assist seniors develop and maintain the physical strength required to do these activities independently.

Regular chair exercises can help older persons improve their functional fitness, which is the capacity to complete daily chores safely and independently. This can give them more confidence in their actions, lessening their fear of falling or being wounded. As a result, chair exercises help seniors age in place by allowing them to stay in their homes and communities for longer periods without requiring considerable assistance.

Furthermore, the enhanced mobility and strength obtained from chair exercises can help seniors enjoy social events, travel, and pursue hobbies, thus improving their quality of life. This sense of independence benefits elders not just physically but also emotionally, allowing them to keep their dignity and autonomy.

9. Mental Health and Cognitive Benefits

While the physical benefits of chair exercises are obvious, the impact on mental health should not be underestimated. Regular physical activity, even modest chair exercises, has been demonstrated to alleviate symptoms of anxiety, melancholy, and stress. Exercise causes the release of endorphins, which are natural mood boosters that improve emotions of well-being. Chair exercises can help seniors who are more prone to emotions of loneliness or isolation.

Chair exercises not only improve mental wellness but also provide cognitive benefits. Many of the movements in chair exercises demand coordination and focus, which can stimulate and improve cognitive function. Exercises that entail lifting the legs while moving the arms, for example, require participants to focus on coordinating numerous movements at the same time, which improves mental clarity.

This cognitive stimulation is especially crucial for the elderly, as regular mental activity can halt cognitive decline and improve memory. Chair exercises, when combined with attentive breathing and intentional movement, can act as a sort of moving meditation, encouraging relaxation and stress reduction. For seniors who suffer from sleep difficulties or high levels of stress, including chair exercises in their regimen can provide both physical and mental relaxation, thereby enhancing their overall quality of life.

10. Promotes Social Interaction and Group Participation

Chair exercises can be done alone, although they are most commonly conducted in groups, such as community centers, senior living facilities, or online exercise programs. This social part of chair exercises has an added benefit because it stimulates interaction and connection with others. Many seniors believe that remaining socially involved is critical to their mental and emotional health. Group exercise environments promote a sense of camaraderie and support, which helps individuals stay motivated and accountable in their fitness regimens.

Exercising with others can also create a lively and enjoyable environment, enhancing the experience and lessening feelings of isolation. Chair exercise courses provide an opportunity for seniors who live alone or far away from family to meet new people, form friendships, and share experiences. This social involvement helps to reduce feelings of loneliness, which can lead to improved mental health.

Even if you prefer to exercise at home, virtual chair exercise sessions or online groups can help you feel more connected and encouraged. Joining a virtual club allows individuals to stay connected and inspired while also exercising in the comfort of their own homes. These cultures encourage camaraderie and shared goals, which can make chair workouts more pleasurable and sustainable as part of a healthy lifestyle.

11. Easy to Modify and Personalize

Another significant advantage of chair exercises is their ease of modification and personalization to meet the needs and goals of each individual. Whether someone is new to exercising or has been active for years, chair exercises provide a versatile framework that can be tailored to fitness level, physical constraints, and personal preferences.

Individuals with joint pain or mobility concerns, for example, might adhere to milder, low-impact activities that emphasize flexibility and mobility, whilst more advanced participants can increase the intensity with resistance bands, weights, or more dynamic routines. This versatility means that chair workouts can continue to challenge and benefit people as their fitness levels improve.

Chair exercises can be designed to target specific health issues, such as improving posture, relieving back pain, or strengthening core muscles. This adjustability makes chair exercises an extremely versatile alternative for anyone trying to achieve specific fitness goals without putting unnecessary strain on their body. Chair workouts encourage a sense of autonomy and self-empowerment in fitness by allowing people to tailor the exercises to their specific needs.

Chair workouts have various specific benefits, making them a good choice for people of all fitness levels, particularly seniors and those with mobility issues. Chair exercises are beneficial for a variety of reasons, including accessibility, safety, adaptability, and convenience. Chair exercises enable people to keep their independence, improve their physical and mental health, and live a healthier lifestyle by providing a low-impact, effective technique to build strength, flexibility, and general fitness.

Physical And Mental Health Advantages

Chair exercises are a unique and effective technique for seniors to engage in physical activity, particularly those who have limited mobility or balance concerns. These activities can dramatically improve physical health, and emotional well-being, and lead to a healthier lifestyle. Below, we'll look at the primary physical and mental health benefits of chair exercises, with a focus on seniors.

Physical Health Benefits:

1. **Increased Strength and Endurance:** One of the key benefits of chair workouts is increased muscular strength and endurance. Regular chair exercises can help seniors improve muscle tone, particularly in the upper and lower body. Exercises that target key muscle groups, such as sitting bicep curls, chest presses, and leg lifts, can help seniors maintain functional strength. This is essential for everyday tasks such as standing up from a chair, climbing stairs, and lifting groceries.

2. **Increased Flexibility:** Flexibility decreases with age, resulting in stiffness and a higher risk of injury. Chair exercises include stretching movements that can improve flexibility in important regions like the back, hips, and shoulders. Poses such as the seated forward bend and seated

twists assist seniors retain their range of motion, allowing them to do daily duties more comfortably.

3. **Enhanced Balance and Coordination:** Falls are a major worry for elders, with many resulting in serious injuries. Chair workouts can enhance balance and coordination by challenging stability. Exercises such as seated leg lifts and side reaches improve core stability, which is necessary for balance. Seniors who do these motions daily can lower their risk of falling and improve their general stability.

4. **Weight Management:** Regular physical exercise, especially when seated, is essential for weight management. Chair exercises can enhance calorie expenditure, which is beneficial for seniors who want to reduce weight or maintain a healthy weight. More dynamic workouts, such as seated marching or leg extensions, can increase the heart rate and aid in weight loss attempts. Maintaining a healthy weight also lowers your risk of developing chronic conditions like diabetes and heart disease.

5. **Cardiovascular Health:** Chair workouts increase cardiovascular fitness by raising the heart rate and boosting circulation. Simple activities, such as seated marches and arm circles, can raise the heart rate and improve cardiovascular health. Regular participation in these activities can help lower blood pressure, improve cholesterol levels, and minimize the risk of heart disease.

6. **Joint Health and Pain Relief:** Many seniors experience joint pain and stiffness, which are commonly caused by illnesses like arthritis. Chair exercises can give mild movements that help to lubricate the joints and enhance overall joint health. Seated stretching and low-impact activities can help seniors manage pain and stiffness, improving their quality of life. Regular mobility is essential for preserving joint function and can assist in alleviating the intensity of arthritis symptoms.

Mental Health Benefits

1. **Reduced Symptoms of Depression and Anxiety:** Physical activity, including chair exercises, has been shown to improve mental health. Regular exercise can release endorphins, the body's natural mood lifters, resulting in fewer feelings of despair and anxiety. Chair exercises might assist elders improve their mood and decrease feelings of loneliness or sadness.

2. **Enhanced Cognitive Function:** There is an increasing amount of evidence indicating that physical activity can improve cognitive performance in older persons. Regular exercise boosts blood flow to the brain, which promotes the formation of new brain cells and improves neuroplasticity. Chair exercises can be an effective tool for seniors because they engage not just the body but also the mind, particularly

when physical activities are combined with memory tasks or coordination challenges.

3. **Enhanced Self-Esteem and Confidence:** Completing chair exercises successfully can provide a sense of accomplishment while also increasing self-esteem and confidence. As seniors improve their strength, flexibility, and balance via exercise, they may feel more capable of partaking in daily tasks. This increased confidence can have a knock-on impact, encouraging individuals to try new activities, mingle more, and participate in community events.

4. **Social Interaction and Connection:** Many senior citizens find inspiration and fun in group chair exercise programs. These social situations allow people to interact with one another, creating a sense of belonging and community. Physical activity with others can lessen emotions of isolation and loneliness, resulting in better mental health. Group sessions also provide a supportive environment in which elders may encourage one another, discuss their experiences, and celebrate their achievements together.

5. **Stress Reduction and Relaxation:** Regular physical activity, such as chair exercises, is a good approach to alleviating stress. Exercise increases the release of neurotransmitters that assist regulate mood, lowering tension and anxiety. Furthermore, chair exercises might include

breathing techniques that encourage relaxation, assisting elders in managing stress levels. Focusing on movement and breathing can be a sort of mindfulness that helps elders center themselves and find peace in the face of daily challenges.

6. **Improved Quality of Life:** Chair exercises provide both physical and mental health advantages, resulting in an improved quality of life. As seniors gain strength, flexibility, and confidence, they may find it easier to participate in social events, pursue hobbies, and live life to the fullest. Regular exercise can provide seniors with the empowerment they need to live a happier and active lifestyle, allowing them to remain independent for longer.

Chair exercises provide several physical and mental health benefits to seniors, making them a valuable supplement to any workout plan. These activities benefit seniors' independence and well-being by improving their strength, flexibility, balance, and cardiovascular health. Furthermore, the mental health benefits, such as reduced depressive symptoms, improved cognitive function, and increased social engagement, highlight the overall benefits of regular physical activity.

For seniors seeking to enhance their health, chair exercises are a safe, effective, and pleasurable approach to stay active and prosper in their golden years. As more elders realize the benefits of chair exercises, they can have healthier, happier, and more rewarding lives.

Impact On Weight Management

Weight control is an important part of maintaining overall health, particularly for seniors over the age of 70. As we age, our metabolism slows, making it more difficult to maintain a healthy weight. Regular physical activity, especially chair exercises, can have a significant impact on weight management.

Weight management entails maintaining a healthy body weight through a combination of nutrition and physical activity. Weight control is especially important for seniors because being overweight increases the risk of chronic diseases like diabetes, heart disease, and joint difficulties. Being underweight, on the other hand, might result in muscle weakness, malnutrition, and impaired immune function. Thus, achieving the appropriate balance is critical.

How Chair Exercises Help Weight Management

1. **Caloric Expenditure:** One of the most effective weight-management strategies is to burn more calories than you ingest. While chair exercises burn fewer calories than high-impact activities, they can still contribute significantly to total caloric expenditure. Seated marching, leg lifts, and upper body motions all activate muscles and raise the heart rate, resulting in calorie burn. Chair exercises are a safe and

effective technique for seniors to increase their physical activity without overdoing it.

2. **Building Muscle Mass:** Sarcopenia is the natural decline of muscle mass with aging. Lower muscle mass might cause a slower metabolism, making it more difficult to keep a healthy weight. Chair exercises that emphasize strength training, such as sitting bicep curls and chest presses, aid in muscle mass development and maintenance. Increased muscle mass not only helps you burn more calories at rest, but it also improves your entire body composition, resulting in a healthy weight.

3. **Improving Metabolism:** Regular physical activity, especially chair exercises, can help improve metabolic function. Exercise increases metabolic pathways that aid in the breakdown of fat and glucose, resulting in a more effective metabolism. This is especially useful for seniors, as a faster metabolic rate can aid in weight loss or management, lowering the risk of weight-related health problems.

4. **Increasing Physical Activity Levels:** Chair exercises might serve as a springboard to more physical activity. For seniors who may have been sedentary, starting with chair exercises can build confidence and stamina, enabling them to engage in more activities outside of their exercise program. As elders acquire strength and mobility, they may be inspired to

try new forms of physical activity, so boosting their weight management efforts.

5. **Accessibility and Sustainability:** One of the major benefits of chair exercises is their convenience. Many seniors may have mobility issues or persistent pain, which can make typical exercises difficult. Chair workouts can be done at home, making it easier to stick to a schedule. The ease with which these exercises can be incorporated into daily life promotes commitment to a consistent workout routine, which is critical for weight management.

Chair exercises can help people over the age of 70 maintain their weight effectively. Seniors who incorporate these simple activities into their daily regimen can increase calorie expenditure, muscle mass, metabolism, and total physical activity levels. When paired with a nutritious diet and attentive eating habits, chair exercises can help seniors reach and maintain a healthy weight, resulting in enhanced overall health and well-being. The path to good weight control may be difficult, but with determination, support, and the correct tools, seniors can successfully traverse this critical element of their health.

Safety Measures And Advice For Seniors

Maintaining physical activity as we age is critical for improving our health, independence, and quality of life. However, prioritizing safety is critical for preventing injuries and ensuring a great experience. The following are thorough safety precautions and advice for elders participating in chair exercises.

1. Consult with a Healthcare Professional

Before beginning any new fitness regimen, seniors should contact their healthcare provider. A doctor or physical therapist can evaluate an individual's health, medications, and physical ability, and provide tailored recommendations on appropriate exercises and any necessary modifications. This phase is critical for seniors with chronic diseases including arthritis, heart disease, or balance problems.

2. Choose the Right Chair

The chair used for workouts should be solid and well-made, preferably without wheels. Here are some crucial variables to consider:

❖ **Height:** The chair should allow the senior's feet to rest flat on the ground while seated. This promotes correct posture and balance.

❖ **Back Support:** A chair with a high back offers support and stability when exercising. It helps reduce back strain and increase comfort.

❖ **Armrests:** Chairs with armrests can help people with limited strength sit and get up more easily.

3. Maintain a Safe Environment

Creating a safe training environment is critical to avoiding falls and injuries. Here are some suggestions to consider:

❖ **Clear the Area:** Remove any clutter, loose rugs, or impediments from the area around the chair to reduce tripping hazards.

❖ **Adequate Lighting:** Make sure the workout space is well-lit to increase visibility and safety. Consider employing strong, natural lighting or overhead lights to illuminate the entire area.

❖ **Non-Slip Flooring:** If feasible, exercise on surfaces that are not slippery. If using a carpet, make sure it is securely tied to the floor.

4. Dress Appropriately

Wearing appropriate attire and footwear can have a big impact on comfort and safety during chair workouts. Here's what you should consider:

- ❖ **Comfortable Clothing:** Wear loose-fitting clothes that allow for unfettered mobility. Avoid anything that restricts movement, such as tight pants or lengthy gowns that could become caught.
- ❖ **Footwear:** Wear supportive, nonslip shoes with good traction. Avoid wearing slippers or flip-flops, as these can increase the chance of slipping.

5. Warm Up and Cool Down

Warming up and cooling down are important parts of any fitness routine, particularly for seniors.

- ❖ **Warm-Up:** A 5-10 minute warm-up regimen gets the body ready for a workout. Gentle motions like seated marches, shoulder rolls, and wrist circles can help enhance blood flow to muscles and joints.
- ❖ **Cool Down:** After finishing the chair exercises, stretch for a few minutes and allow your heart rate to gradually decline. This helps to avoid muscular soreness and increases flexibility.

6. Listen to Your Body

Seniors should be aware of their bodies and understand the importance of listening to how they feel during exercise.

- ❖ **Stop if in Pain:** If any workout produces discomfort or pain, you must stop immediately. Pain is typically an indication that something is wrong, and continuing may result in harm.
- ❖ **Modify Exercises:** Not every workout will be appropriate for everyone. Seniors should feel free to adapt routines to suit their comfort level. For example, if a leg lift is too difficult, a sitting leg slide may be a preferable alternative.

7. Stay Hydrated

Proper hydration is essential for everyone, but it's especially crucial for seniors, who may not feel thirsty even when their bodies require fluids.

Take Water Before and After: Encourage elders to take a glass of water before beginning their exercise program, and then hydrate again afterward. If your workout lasts more than an hour, it's best to stay hydrated.

8. Practice Proper Breathing Techniques

Breathing appropriately during exercise can improve performance and safety.

Seniors should breathe deeply and steadily during their workouts. Inhale via the nose during easy workouts and exhale through the mouth during more difficult ones. This method helps to provide oxygen to the muscles and promotes relaxation.

9. Incorporate Balance Exercises

Chair exercises can be coupled with balance training to increase stability and lower the chance of falling.

Including simple balance movements in your routine, such as seated heel-to-toe movements or leg raises, will help to strengthen the core and improve stability. Over time, these activities might make seniors feel more safe and confident while standing or walking.

10. Encourage Social Interaction

Exercises performed with others can bring motivation, encouragement, and fun.

Consider attending a chair exercise class at your local community center or gym. Exercising with others promotes a sense of community and might increase accountability.

Invite family members to join in the exercises, making it an enjoyable activity that develops connections while boosting health.

11. Track Your Progress

Keeping track of progress can be an effective motivation for seniors.

Encourage elders to keep an activity notebook in which they can record the types of activities they do, the time of each, and how they feel afterward. This record can be used to track progress over time and encourage people to stay engaged.

12. Seek Professional Guidance

Seeking professional advice can be quite beneficial for those who are new to exercise or are unclear on how to proceed safely.

Consult a professional trainer who specializes in senior fitness, or a physical therapist. They can create tailored exercise routines that ensure motions are done safely and successfully.

Chair exercises can help elders maintain good physical health, improve their quality of life, and regain independence. Safety should always be the highest consideration. Following these precautions and advice will allow seniors to enjoy a safe and successful fitness regimen that suits their specific demands and improves their well-being.

Equipment And Tools Required For Chair Exercises

When going on a path to increase physical fitness with chair exercises, having the proper equipment and tools can greatly boost the effectiveness of your regimen. While many chair exercises may be done without any specialist equipment, a few basic items can help make workouts more comfortable, safe, and fun. This section will go over crucial equipment and tools that can help seniors with their chair exercise regimens.

1. A Sturdy Chair

The most basic piece of equipment for chair workouts is a solid chair. This chair should be solid, comfy, and suited to the user's height. Here are some important considerations:

The chair should be designed so that the user may sit with their feet flat on the ground, knees bent at a 90-degree angle, and hips somewhat higher than the knees. This stance is essential for maintaining correct posture and balance while exercising.

Armrests can provide extra support, making it easier to get in and out of a chair. A chair with a straight back promotes proper posture, which is required for various workouts.

Make sure the chair has a non-slip surface or is placed on a sturdy floor to avoid slipping while moving.

2. Resistance Bands

Resistance bands are useful and inexpensive instruments that provide resistance to chair workouts, thus increasing strength and endurance. They come in a variety of resistance levels, making them appropriate for users of varying fitness levels. When utilizing resistance bands, consider the following.

Types include loop bands, flat bands, and tube bands. Loop bands are generally more convenient for seated workouts since they may be fastened under the feet, whereas tube bands include handles for improved grip.

Resistance bands can be used for a wide range of exercises, including seated bicep curls, chest presses, and leg lifts. They offer a safe technique to build resistance without the risk of harm that comes with large weights.

3. Light Dumbbells

Light dumbbells are another useful supplement to a chair training regimen. They are great for strengthening the upper body and may be used in several activities. Here's something to remember:

Select a weight that is both manageable and difficult. For seniors, this could range from 1 to 5 pounds, depending on their strength capabilities.

Grip: Choose dumbbells with a comfortable grip. Some may feature rubberized or textured surfaces to prevent slippage, which is especially helpful for people with limited hand strength.

Use dumbbells that do not create strain or discomfort. Starting with lesser weights and progressively increasing as strength improves is recommended.

4. Yoga Mat or Nonslip Surface

Using a yoga mat or ensuring a non-slip surface can improve the safety of chair workouts. A mat cushions the feet and prevents slips and falls. Consider the following.

A thicker mat can give additional padding, making it more suitable for seated activities.

Place the mat on a stable, flat surface to prevent movement during workouts.

5. Chair Yoga Block or Pillow

A yoga block or firm pillow can help provide support and comfort during a variety of movements. Here's how they can be used.

A block or pillow can be used to elevate the legs during specific stretches, making movements easier to do.

They can also provide additional support during seated activities, allowing you to maintain appropriate posture.

Using a pillow with a firm construction might improve comfort during long workouts.

6. Water Bottle

Staying hydrated is essential for any exercise routine, even chair exercises. Keeping a water bottle handy serves various purposes:

Keeping water widely accessible encourages frequent hydration breaks.

A lightweight, portable water bottle allows you to keep hydrated during your workout.

7. Towel

A towel can serve various tasks during chair workouts.

Placing a towel over the chair seat might provide extra comfort and support when seated.

A towel can also be used to wipe sweat and keep hygiene during workouts, particularly in warmer climates.

8. Music or Audio Device

Using music or an audio device can make chair exercises more pleasurable and encouraging. Here are a few reasons why you should consider this tool.

Upbeat music helps fuel workouts, increasing mood and motivation.

Guided audio workouts can provide instruction and timing, making it easier for elders to complete exercises.

9. Exercise Guide or Video Resource

Having access to an exercise guide or video resource can greatly improve the chair exercise experience. Consider the following.

Visual instruction can help ensure that exercises are done correctly, lowering the chance of injury.

Resources that include a range of activities help keep routines interesting and engaging, promoting frequent involvement.

Many guides feature tracking tools to help you create and achieve your goals.

10. Supportive Footwear

While not considered equipment in the traditional sense, proper footwear is essential for safety and comfort during chair workouts. Here are a few tips:

Shoes with non-slip soles help minimize falls, especially while rising or getting out of a chair.

Properly fitted shoes give proper support and comfort, lowering the likelihood of discomfort during exercise.

Equipping oneself with the proper equipment for chair exercises can improve the overall experience, making sessions safer and more successful. A solid chair, resistance bands, light dumbbells, and other supportive items not only give diversity to workout routines but also address the specific needs of elders. By providing a comfortable and safe atmosphere, seniors can participate more fully in their exercise regimens, resulting in improved physical fitness, greater independence, and a higher quality of life. As usual, before beginning any new exercise regimen, contact a healthcare physician, especially if you have pre-existing health concerns.

CHAPTER 2: GETTING STARTED WITH YOUR EXERCISE ROUTINE

Evaluate Your Current Fitness Level

Assessing your present fitness level is an important first step in creating an efficient exercise plan, particularly for seniors over 70. Understanding your current physical health can help you set realistic objectives, customize your training routine to your ability, and track your progress over time. This assessment can also alert your healthcare professional to any unique limits you may have.

Why should you assess your fitness level?

1. **Personalized Approach:** Everyone's body is different, especially as we age. Assessing your fitness level allows you to tailor your training regimen to your specific goals and restrictions.

2. **Identifying Strengths and limitations:** Knowing your strengths can help you grow on them while acknowledging your limitations can direct you to areas for progress.

3. **Goal Setting:** By evaluating your fitness level, you can set realistic goals that will inspire you without overwhelming you.

4. **Tracking Progress:** Regular assessments can help you measure your progress over time, giving you inspiration and a sense of success.

5. **Injury Prevention:** An accurate examination identifies potential health risks or injuries, allowing you to avoid exercises that may aggravate pre-existing conditions.

When evaluating your fitness level, examine the following major areas:

❖ **Cardiovascular Endurance:** This refers to your heart and lung's ability to withstand physical exertion over time.

   One basic way is the Timed Walk Test. Find a flat, straight path (such as a corridor or track) and see how far you can walk in six minutes. For seniors, a distance of 300-400 meters is typical. If you have a stationary bike or treadmill, you can use it instead.

❖ **Muscular Strength:** Muscular strength is the maximum amount of force that a muscle can generate.

You can do a Chair Stand Test. Sit on the edge of a sturdy chair, arms folded over your chest. Stand up and then sit down for 30 seconds. Count how many times you can stand up in that timeframe. A decent score is usually between 8 and 12 repetitions. For a more advanced test, evaluate your ability to perform sitting bicep curls with light weights.

❖ **Flexibility:** Flexibility is the range of motion in your joints and muscles.

The Chair Sit and Reach Test is an excellent alternative. Sit on the edge of a chair and extend one leg straight out in front of you, keeping the other foot on the floor. With both hands, reach for your toes on the extended leg. Determine how far you can stretch past your toes. A distance of 2-4 inches past your toes is regarded as appropriate for elders.

❖ **Balance is essential for avoiding falls and retaining independence.**

The Single Leg Stand Test can be performed using a chair for support. Stand on one leg for as long as possible without touching anything. Ideally, aim for at least 10 seconds per leg.

❖ **Body Composition:** What It Is. Body composition is the proportion of fat and non-fat mass in your body.

While the most precise measurements necessitate specialist equipment, simple approaches such as measuring your waist circumference can suffice. A waist circumference of more than 35 inches for women and 40 inches for males may suggest an increased risk of health issues.

Tools for Assessment

- ❖ **Fitness Trackers:** Wearable fitness trackers can provide useful information about your daily activity levels, heart rate, and sleep habits, all of which contribute to your overall fitness level.

- ❖ **Mobile Apps:** There are numerous apps available that can assist you navigate assessments and track your progress over time.

- ❖ **Professional Assessment:** If possible, consult with a personal trainer or physical therapist who specializes in senior fitness. They can do a thorough evaluation and design a personalized training program based on your requirements.

Assessing your present fitness level is an important step in developing an efficient exercise plan for your needs as a senior. Understanding your cardiovascular endurance, muscular strength, flexibility, balance, and body composition allows you to create realistic objectives, track your progress, and ultimately enhance your overall health and well-being. Remember that the route to fitness is unique to each individual, and you must proceed at your own pace.

Setting Achievable Goals And Tracking Progress

To reap the full advantages of chair exercises, it is critical to set realistic goals and track progress efficiently. Setting objectives is an important part of any workout regimen since it gives direction and inspiration. Goals help you focus on your objectives, making it easier to create a disciplined plan of action. Well-defined goals for elders doing chair exercises can result in better physical health, more confidence, and a higher quality of life.

Goals can be divided into two categories: short-term and long-term.

Short-term goals can be achieved in a matter of weeks or months. They can serve as stepping stones to larger goals and help you stay motivated.

Long-term goals are more significant and can take months or even years to complete. These objectives provide a larger perspective for your fitness journey, allowing you to focus on significant milestones.

When creating goals, especially for chair exercises, make sure they're reasonable, attainable, and appropriate for your skills. *Here's a step-by-step guide for effective goal setting:*

1. Consider your strength, flexibility, balance, and general mobility. This examination will assist you in determining what is achievable and establishing acceptable goals.

2. Consider which parts of your fitness you'd like to improve. Do you wish to gain strength, and flexibility, lose weight, or improve your balance? Identifying distinct areas of focus will allow you to set more focused goals.

3. Set SMART goals. To ensure the effectiveness of your goals, apply the SMART criteria:

    * ***Specific:*** Identify your goals (for example, "I want to improve my leg strength").
    * ***Measurable:*** Create criteria to track your progress (for example, "I will be able to perform 10 seated leg lifts in a row").
    * ***Achievable:*** Make sure your goals are reasonable for your present fitness level and any constraints (e.g., "I will increase my seated leg lifts from 5 to 10 within four weeks").
    * ***Relevant:*** Your goals should be consistent with your overall health aims (for example, "Improving my strength will help me maintain independence").
    * ***Time:*** Set a time limit for attaining your goals (for example, "I will complete this within the next month").

4. Life can be unpredictable, therefore it's important to be adaptive. If you have difficulties or setbacks, reassess your objectives and alter them as necessary. Flexibility helps keep you engaged and devoted to your training regimen.

Tracking Your Progress

Once you've set your goals, tracking your progress is essential for staying motivated and on track. Monitoring your achievements allows you to appreciate successes while also identifying areas that may require further focus. *Here are some excellent strategies for tracking progress:*

1. Record your workouts, repetitions, and feelings during each session. Recording this information will allow you to see your progress over time and gain insight into your accomplishments.

2. Create a Progress Chart to visually track your goals and progress. You can use charts or graphs to keep track of specific metrics like the number of repetitions or exercise duration. Visual aids can be very encouraging and show you how far you've gone.

3. Divide your long-term goals into smaller, more attainable steps. Celebrate your accomplishments when you hit each

milestone, whether it's increasing your performance in a certain activity or being consistent with your program.

4. Regularly review your fitness journey. Consider how your goals have changed, the problems you've faced, and how your body feels. Reflection can provide vital insights and allow you to change your goals as needed.

5. Share your goals and successes with family and friends for support and accountability. Having a support system can increase your motivation and help you stick to your fitness plan.

Setting realistic objectives and tracking progress are essential components of a successful fitness routine for seniors who participate in chair exercises. By measuring your current fitness level, identifying specific areas for development, and defining goals using the SMART criteria, you may chart a clear road to reaching your fitness goals. Tracking your progress using a fitness notebook, charts, and milestones will help you stay motivated and accountable.

Creating A Weekly Exercise Plan

Creating a structured weekly exercise plan is essential for seniors looking to improve their health and maintain mobility. A well-designed plan provides a roadmap to achieve fitness goals, enhances accountability, and promotes consistency.

A. Frequency and Duration

Frequency: Aim for at least 150 minutes of moderate-intensity exercise per week, as recommended by health authorities. For seniors, this can be broken down into shorter sessions spread throughout the week. For example, aim for 30 minutes of exercise five times a week.

Duration: Each session should include time for warm-up, main exercises, and cool-down. A typical session might look like this:
Warm-up: 5 minutes
Main exercises: 20-25 minutes
Cool-down: 5-10 minutes

B. Exercise Types

Incorporate a variety of exercise types into your weekly plan to address different aspects of fitness:

1. **Strength Training:** Include 2-3 days of strength training exercises focused on major muscle groups. For example, chair exercises such as seated bicep curls, seated shoulder presses, and modified chair squats can help build muscle and maintain bone density.

2. **Cardiovascular Exercise:** Aim for 2-3 days of cardiovascular exercise to improve heart health and stamina. This could involve chair marching, seated jacks, or even brisk walking if you feel comfortable. Remember to start slow and gradually increase intensity.

3. **Flexibility and Balance Exercises:** Dedicate time for flexibility and balance exercises at least 2-3 days a week. Seated stretches, seated tree poses, and other stretching routines enhance flexibility and help prevent falls.

Here's a sample weekly exercise plan tailored for seniors:

Day	Activity	Duration
Monday	Strength training (e.g., bicep curls)	30 mins
Tuesday	Cardiovascular exercise (seated marching)	30 mins
Wednesday	Flexibility exercises (e.g., seated stretches)	30 mins
Thursday	Strength training (e.g., chair squats)	30 mins
Friday	Cardiovascular exercise (seated jacks)	30 mins
Saturday	Flexibility and balance (e.g., tree pose)	30 mins
Sunday	Rest day or gentle walk	-

Feel free to adjust the plan based on your preferences and schedule, you could as well come up with a structure that best fits your schedule. The key is to find a routine that works for you and keeps you engaged.

While structure is important, it's equally vital to remain flexible with your exercise plan. Life can be unpredictable, and it's okay to modify your routine based on how you feel each day. If you're not up for a full workout, consider doing a shorter session or focusing on gentle stretches instead. The goal is to maintain an active lifestyle without adding unnecessary stress.

Creating a weekly exercise plan is a powerful tool for seniors seeking to improve their health and maintain independence. By assessing your fitness level as discussed earlier in previous sections, setting realistic goals, and structuring a balanced routine, you can make significant strides toward better health. Remember to track your progress, incorporate social aspects, and stay flexible to ensure that your exercise journey remains enjoyable and sustainable. With commitment and consistency, you can enhance your quality of life and embrace the benefits of regular physical activity.

Incorporating Social Aspects Into Chair Exercise Routines

Physical activity is vital for maintaining good health, especially for seniors over the age of 70. As people face the challenges of aging, including social features in exercise regimens can significantly improve motivation, adherence, and general well-being. Group sessions, family participation, and social interactions build a sense of belonging, accountability, and encouragement, which can have a huge impact on their fitness journey.

Importance of Social Interaction during Exercise

Social involvement is an essential human requirement. It is especially important for elders, who may feel isolated or lonely. Participating in group exercise courses or incorporating family members in fitness routines might help to establish a positive environment that combats negative thoughts. According to research, seniors who participate in social activities are more likely to continue their fitness routines and reap the numerous physical and mental health benefits that regular physical activity provides.

1. **Increased Motivation:** Exercising with others can enhance motivation. Participants in a group environment can support one another, share obstacles, and enjoy victories together.

This shared experience might motivate elders to push through discomfort or tiredness, knowing they have a support system behind them.

2. **Increased Accountability:** Group classes or family involvement can encourage accountability. When seniors know that others expect them to attend a lesson or complete an exercise session, they are less inclined to skip it. This dedication to others can provide them with the motivation they need to stay consistent.

3. **Improved Mental Well-Being:** Socializing while exercising can help elders overcome emotions of loneliness and sadness. Conversations, sharing experiences, and developing connections in a social context can improve mood and mental health.

Group Classes

Group exercise programs designed specifically for seniors are a fantastic way to add social features to chair exercise regimens. These sessions are often led by qualified instructors who understand the unique needs of older persons and can adapt workouts to different fitness levels.

1. **Available Sessions:** Community centers, gyms, and senior living facilities offer a variety of chair exercise sessions. *Options could include:*

* ***Chair Yoga:*** This is a mild style of yoga that encourages flexibility, balance, and relaxation while seated.
* ***Chair Aerobics:*** It is a high-energy session that focuses on improving cardiovascular fitness and strength via rhythmic exercises while seated.
* ***Strength Training Classes:*** These programs, which focus on muscle strength, generally use resistance bands or light weights while seated.

2. **Establishing a Community:** Regular attendance at group programs encourages individuals to build ties with their peers. Over time, these interactions can develop into friendships, giving social support outside of the workout setting. Seniors may look forward to lessons not only for the exercise but also for the camaraderie they share with their classmates.

3. **Engaging Instructors:** Skilled instructors not only direct exercises but also foster an inclusive environment. They can facilitate group discussions, provide ideas, and incorporate social components into classrooms. An engaging instructor can encourage learners to interact with one another, creating a sense of community.

Family Participation

Involving family members in chair exercise routines can greatly increase a senior's motivation and enjoyment. Exercise becomes a shared activity that promotes bonding, develops long-term memories, and strengthens family bonds.

1. **Establishing a Family Exercise Routine:** Family members can plan regular exercise sessions with their elderly loved ones, making it an enjoyable and engaging part of their daily routine. Whether it's a weekly chair exercise class or a home workout, this shared commitment strengthens family relationships and promotes healthy behaviors for future generations.

2. **Making It Fun:** Family engagement does not have to be limited to formal exercise. Fun activities, such as dance parties, movement-based games, or simply a light walk in the park, can help seniors stay involved while also encouraging physical exercise. The aim is to maintain the environment lighthearted and entertaining.

3. **Fostering Understanding and Support:** Family members can learn about the precise activities that assist their elderly loved ones, allowing them to grasp the value of physical activity in sustaining health and independence. This information can lead to increased empathy and support,

making it simpler for seniors to stick to their exercise schedules.

4. **Developing Healthy Habits:** Seniors can set a good example for future generations by including their families in fitness. This contact can encourage family members to lead more active lifestyles, supporting overall family wellness.

Overcoming Barriers to Social Participation

While the benefits of including social aspects in exercise are obvious, some seniors may find barriers to participation. Addressing these hurdles is critical to creating an inclusive and supportive atmosphere.

1. **Transportation Issues:** Many seniors may struggle to get to group programs or community centers. Family members might assist by offering rides or organizing workout sessions at home. Community initiatives may also provide transportation for seniors to attend classes.

2. **Health Concerns:** Seniors may be concerned about their health and capacity to participate in group workouts. It is critical to ensure that lessons are delivered by qualified teachers who can modify exercises to different skill levels. Family members can also advise seniors to speak with their healthcare providers before beginning any new fitness regimen.

3. **Fear of Judgment:** Seniors may be self-conscious of their talents in a group situation. It is critical to foster a welcoming workplace in which everyone is encouraged, regardless of fitness ability. Positive encouragement from teachers and other participants might assist in reducing these worries.

4. **Lack of Awareness:** Some seniors may be unaware of the various alternatives for group classes or family involvement in exercise. Community outreach programs, flyers in local centers, and word-of-mouth from family and friends can all contribute to increased knowledge of available options.

Incorporating social features into chair exercise routines is an effective strategy to improve the fitness experience for seniors over the age of 70. Seniors can discover inspiration, accountability, and a sense of belonging by participating in group classes and with their families. They can celebrate their triumphs and overcome problems with others, resulting in better physical health and general well-being. Seniors who build social relationships can make their fitness regimens more fun, sustainable, and a vital part of their lives.

CHAPTER 3: WARM-UP EXERCISES

The Importance Of Warming Up

Warming up is a crucial part of any exercise regimen, especially for seniors who participate in chair exercises. It involves gradually boosting heart rate, blood flow, and muscle temperature in order to prepare the body for physical exertion. This preparatory period not only improves performance but also minimizes the likelihood of harm. Below, we'll go over the importance of warming up, its advantages, and how to include it in your exercise regimen.

1. Physiological Benefits

❖ **Increased Blood Flow and Oxygen Supply:** As you warm up, your heart rate rises, pumping more blood around your body. This increased blood flow provides more oxygen and nutrients to the muscles, which is necessary for peak performance. Muscles become more efficient in creating energy as they absorb adequate oxygen, enabling longer periods of exercise. Warming up is especially important for seniors who may have limited circulation since it ensures their bodies can tolerate physical exertion safely.

❖ **Enhanced Muscle Temperature:** Warming up raises muscle temperature, which is necessary for muscle flexibility and overall function. Warmer muscles are more flexible, which reduces stiffness and increases joint range of motion. This is especially useful for seniors, who may have stiffness owing to age-related changes in their muscles and connective tissues. Warming up can improve the effectiveness and comfort of chair exercises for seniors by increasing flexibility.

2. Injury Prevention

❖ **Reducing Muscular Strain:** One of the most serious consequences of exercising without warming up is muscular strain. Cold muscles are more prone to injuries like pulls and tears, which can be especially dangerous for the elderly. Seniors can reduce their risk of injury by gradually increasing the intensity of their activities through warm-ups.

❖ **Joint Lubrication:** Warming up promotes the creation of synovial fluid, which lubricates joints. This is critical for preserving joint health and function, especially in older persons who may suffer from arthritis or joint pain. Well-lubricated joints can move more freely, which is essential for the effectiveness and safety of chair workouts.

3. Mental Preparation

❖ **Psychological Readiness:** Warming up has both a physical and psychological goal. It allows seniors to mentally prepare for their workouts, shifting their concentration away from daily distractions and onto their health goals. Engaging in light physical activity can also improve mood, making exercise more fun and less daunting.

❖ **Establishing a Routine:** Including a warm-up routine will help you develop a consistent workout habit. It signals to the brain that it is time to participate in physical activity, emphasizing the significance of regular exercise. For seniors who struggle with motivation, a familiar warm-up can make beginning an exercise session more appealing.

Types of Warm-up Exercises

Dynamic stretching entails moving several portions of your body while gradually increasing reach, speed, or both. Examples include arm circles, leg swings, and torso twists. These movements not only improve flexibility but also prepare the body for the specialized motions required in chair exercises.

Light cardiovascular workouts like seated marching, side bends, and soft toe taps will help warm up the body. These activities increase the heart rate and get the blood circulating without placing too much pressure on the body.

Breathing Techniques: Including deep breathing techniques in the warm-up might help to relax the mind and body. Deep breathing enhances oxygen intake and reduces anxiety, establishing a pleasant tone for the upcoming workout.

Recommendations for Seniors

Warm-ups for seniors should take 5 to 10 minutes, with the intensity progressively rising. The idea is to increase heart rate and muscle warmth without overexertion. Begin with low-intensity movements and progressively increase to more dynamic ones.

The warm-up should be tailored to individual fitness levels and any pre-existing health concerns. Seniors should listen to their bodies and make adjustments to avoid discomfort. Seated warm-up activities might be very beneficial for people who have limited mobility.

To gain the full benefits of warming up, seniors should make it a non-negotiable part of their workout regimen. Consistency, like with another workout, is essential for developing strength, flexibility, and general fitness.

Warming up is an important phase in preparing the body for exercise, particularly for seniors who perform chair exercises. A proper warm-up can considerably improve a workout's safety and efficacy by improving blood flow, raising muscle temperature, lowering the chance of injury, and promoting mental preparation. Seniors should make warming up an essential element of their fitness program to ensure they can get the advantages of exercise safely and effectively.

In conclusion, the importance of warming up cannot be emphasized; it provides the cornerstone for a good exercise session, laying the groundwork for better health, mobility, and independence. Seniors who incorporate a complete warm-up regimen can embark on their fitness journeys with confidence and joy, knowing they are making critical efforts to protect their bodies while working toward their health goals.

Simple Warm-Up Routines To Perform While Seated

Warm-up exercises are essential for getting the body ready for more strenuous physical activity, increasing flexibility, and avoiding injuries. Warm-up routines while seated can be a safe and effective strategy for seniors to engage in physical activity, especially those over the age of 70. This strategy allows individuals to get the advantages of exercise while avoiding the risk of falling or discomfort. Below are numerous seated warm-up activities that target different muscle areas, boost circulation, and improve general well-being.

1. Seated Marching

Duration: 2–3 minutes

Seated marching is an effective approach to increase blood flow to the legs and prepare for other workouts.

Instructions:

1. Sit upright in a firm chair, your feet flat on the ground.
2. Begin marching by elevating one knee to your chest and raising the opposing arm.
3. Slowly and steadily alternate sides.
4. Maintain proper posture and take deep breaths.

Benefits: This exercise improves cardiovascular circulation, warms up the hip flexors, and increases coordination.

2. Neck Rolls

Duration: 1–2 minutes

Neck rolls serve to relieve stress in the neck and shoulders, making them a must-do warm-up for anyone who spends time sitting.

Instructions:

1. Sit comfortably, back straight and shoulders relaxed.
2. Gently lower your right ear to your right shoulder.
3. Slowly roll your head forward, allowing your chin to burrow into your chest.
4. Continue to move your head to the left, bringing your left ear near your left shoulder.
5. Reverse the direction and continue the sequence.

Benefits: This routine improves neck mobility, reduces stiffness, and promotes relaxation.

3. Shoulder Rolls

Duration: 1–2 minutes

Shoulder rolls work the shoulder girdle, increasing mobility and decreasing strain.

Instructions:

1. Sit with your back straight and arms relaxed by your sides.
2. Inhale deeply as you raise your shoulders near your ears.
3. Exhale while rolling your shoulders back and down.
4. Repeat 10-15 times, then turn to rolling your shoulders forward.

Benefits: This exercise improves shoulder flexibility, lowers muscle tension, and promotes relaxation.

4. Seated Arm Raises

Duration: 1–2 minutes

Seated arm raises promote blood flow to the upper body and improve shoulder mobility.

Instructions:

1. Sit tall on your chair, feet flat on the floor.

2. Inhale while raising both arms upward, keeping them straight.
3. Exhale while lowering your arms back to your sides.
4. Repeat this motion 10-15 times while focusing on your breathing.

Benefits: This warm-up technique helps to enhance shoulder flexibility and arm strength while exercising the core muscles.

5. Torso Twists

Duration: 1–2 minutes

Torso twists promote spinal mobility and flexibility in the core muscles.

Instructions:

1. Sit up straight with your feet flat on the floor and your hands resting on your knees.
2. Inhale deeply and stretch your spine.
3. As you exhale, slowly twist your torso to the right, resting your left hand on your right knee for support.
4. Hold for a few seconds then return to the center.
5. Repeat on the left side.
6. Do 5-10 twists on each side.

Benefits: This exercise improves spinal flexibility, stimulates digestion, and works the core muscles.

6. Wrist and Ankle Rotations

Duration: 2–3 minutes

Wrist and ankle rotations are essential for warming up joints and increasing mobility.

Instructions:

1. To perform wrist rotations, extend one arm in front of you with the palm pointing downward.
2. Rotate your wrist clockwise for 10-15 seconds before switching to counterclockwise.
3. Repeat on the opposite wrist.
4. Lift one foot slightly off the ground, then rotate your ankle clockwise and counterclockwise for 10-15 seconds. Repeat for the opposite ankle.

Benefits: These movements improve joint flexibility, reduce stiffness, and increase general mobility.

7. Seated Side Bends

Duration: 1–2 minutes

Seated side bends stretch the muscles on the sides of the body, increasing flexibility and reducing tension.

Instructions:

1. Sit tall, with your feet flat on the ground and your hands resting against your thighs.
2. Inhale and raise your right arm overhead.
3. Exhale as you bend to the left and feel a stretch on your right side.
4. Hold for a few seconds and then return to the center.
5. Repeat on the opposite side.
6. Do 5-10 repetitions on each side.

Benefits: This exercise increases flexibility in the spine and oblique muscles, which improves overall mobility.

8. Seated Heel Slides

Duration: 1–2 minutes

Heel slides engage the legs and increase lower body movement without putting stress on the joints.

Instructions:

1. Sit at the edge of your chair, back straight.
2. Extend one leg in front of you while maintaining the heel on the floor.
3. Gently move your heel back toward your body, bending your knee.
4. Repeat the action 10-15 times on each leg.

Benefits: This program improves leg mobility and develops the quadriceps while keeping a safe seated position.

9. Deep Breathing Exercises

Duration: 2–3 minutes

Deep breathing is a vital component of any warm-up regimen since it increases oxygen flow and promotes relaxation.

Instructions:

1. Sit comfortably, hands resting on your knees.
2. Inhale deeply through your nose to fill your lungs and expand your belly.
3. Hold your breath for a moment.
4. Exhale slowly through your lips, letting your body relax.
5. Repeat the method for 5-10 breaths.

Benefits: Deep breathing relaxes the neurological system, decreases tension, and prepares the body for exercise.

Warm-up routines while seated are an important part of fitness, especially for seniors. These basic yet effective exercises help to increase flexibility, and circulation, and prepare the body for more strenuous activity. By including these seated warm-up activities in their daily routine, seniors can get the advantages of physical activity while prioritizing their safety and comfort. Remember to urge participants to listen to their bodies and modify the intensity and duration of the exercises as needed. With constant practice, these warm-ups can have a substantial impact on general health and well-being, encouraging a more active and rewarding lifestyle.

Breathing Strategies To Relax

Breathing is an essential part of our lives, but many people underestimate its importance in both physical and mental health. During times of stress or anxiety, our breathing becomes shallow and fast, exacerbating feelings of tightness and unease. In contrast, using specialized breathing techniques can encourage relaxation, reduce stress, and improve general health. This section will look at a variety of useful breathing techniques that can assist seniors and people of all ages to relax and calm down.

Before getting into specific techniques, it's critical to understand the importance of breath awareness. Breath awareness entails becoming aware of your breathing patterns and understanding how they relate to your mental and physical states. By becoming more aware of your breathing, you can recognize points of stress and intentionally adjust to deeper, more soothing breathing patterns.

Breath awareness can be an effective method for relaxing. *Here are some crucial points to consider:*

❖ Being present and attentive to your breath can help you feel more grounded at the moment, reducing anxiety and overload.

❖ Understanding how your breath changes in response to different emotions might help you gain control over your reactions to stress.
❖ Deep, steady breathing can activate the body's relaxation response, which counteracts the fight-or-flight response caused by stress.

Breathing Techniques for Relaxation

1. Diaphragmatic respiration (belly breathing)

Diaphragmatic breathing, often known as belly breathing, involves drawing air deep into the lungs to increase oxygen absorption. This approach improves relaxation by stimulating the parasympathetic nervous system, which relaxes the body.

How To Practice:

1. Sit or lie in a comfortable position.
2. Place one hand on your chest, and the other on your abdomen.
3. Inhale deeply via your nose, letting your abdomen rise while your chest remains relatively still.
4. Exhale slowly through your lips, feeling your abdomen relax.
5. Repeat for a few minutes, concentrating on the rise and fall of your abdomen.

2. 4-7-8 Breathing

Dr. Andrew Weil developed the 4-7-8 breathing technique, which is intended to relieve anxiety and increase relaxation. This technique consists of inhaling, holding, and exhaling your breath for precise counts.

How To Practice:

1. Start by sitting or sleeping in a comfortable position.
2. Close your eyes and inhale deeply through your nose for a count of four.
3. Hold your breath for the count of seven.
4. Exhale gently and thoroughly through your mouth for a count of eight.
5. Repeat this cycle for four full breaths, increasing the number of repetitions as you get more comfortable.

3. Box Breathing (square breathing)

Box breathing is a simple yet efficient method used by sports and military personnel to improve concentration and reduce stress. This technique involves breathing, holding, exhaling, and holding the breath for equal counts, resulting in a "box" pattern.

How To Practice:

1. Sit comfortably, with your back straight.
2. Inhale deeply through your nose for a count of 4.
3. Hold your breath for 4 counts.
4. Exhale slowly through your mouth for a count of four.
5. Hold your breath again for a count of four.
6. Repeat this cycle for a few minutes, concentrating on the rhythm of your breathing.

4. Nadi Shodhana (alternate nostril breathing)

Nadi Shodhana, or alternating nostril breathing, is a yogic method for balancing the body's energies and calming the mind. This activity can help reduce stress and improve mental clarity.

How To Practice:

1. Sit comfortably, with your spine straight.
2. Use your right thumb to seal your right nostril.
3. Inhale deeply from the left nostril.
4. Close your left nostril with your right ring finger, then release your right nose.
5. Exhale from your right nostril.
6. Inhale deeply through your right nostril and then close it with your thumb.
7. Release your left nostril and breathe through it.

8. Continue this pattern for many minutes, concentrating on the sensations of your breathing.

5. Visualization Breathing

Visualization along with breathing can help to relax you by activating your imagination. This approach allows you to visualize a serene scene while focusing on your breath.

How To Practice:

1. Locate a comfortable position and close your eyes.
2. To find your core, take a few deep breaths.
3. As you inhale, imagine a calming color or environment (such as a peaceful beach or forest).
4. As you exhale, envision releasing tension and stress into the atmosphere.
5. Continue this procedure for a few minutes, allowing yourself to become completely immersed in the visualization.

The use of various breathing techniques provides multiple benefits for relaxation and overall well-being, including:

❖ **Reduced Stress and Anxiety:** Slow, deep breathing activates the parasympathetic nervous system, which lowers cortisol levels and reduces anxiety.

- ❖ **Improved Focus and Concentration:** Mindful breathing methods can improve mental clarity and focus, allowing you to tackle tasks more easily.
- ❖ **Better Sleep Quality:** Including breathing exercises in your nighttime routine will help you relax, making it easier to fall and remain asleep.
- ❖ **Improved Physical Health:** Deep breathing helps increase oxygen flow throughout the body, which benefits cardiovascular health and overall vigor.

To reap the full benefits of these breathing techniques, integrate them into your everyday routine:

- ❖ **Practice in the Morning:** Begin each day with a few minutes of deep breathing to set a pleasant tone.
- ❖ **Use in Stressful Situations:** When you're feeling overwhelmed or stressed, take a moment to practice one of the breathing techniques to help you restore control.
- ❖ **Create a Relaxation Routine:** Set aside time each day for relaxation, combining breathing techniques with other relaxing activities like mild stretching or meditation.

Breathing exercises are an effective way to promote relaxation, reduce stress, and improve general well-being. By implementing these practices into your daily routine, you can develop a stronger sense of calm and resilience, allowing you to negotiate life's problems more easily. Whether you use diaphragmatic breathing, 4-7-8 breathing, box breathing, or another technique, the important is to find what works for you and make it a regular part of your wellness routine.

CHAPTER 4: CHAIR EXERCISES FOR WEIGHT LOSS

1. Seated forward fold pose (Paschimottanasana)

Instructions:

1. Sit on the edge of a sturdy chair, feet level on the floor, hip-width apart.
2. Inhale and extend your arms upwards to lengthen your spine.
3. Exhale and fold forward, bending at the hips and reaching for your feet, shins, or ankles.
4. When leaning forward, keep your spine long to avoid rounding your back.
5. Maintain the position for a few breaths, feeling the stretch in your hamstrings and back.
6. To release, gradually return to an upright position.

Benefits:

- Increases flexibility by stretching the spine, hamstrings, and shoulders.
- Helps to relieve anxiety and stress, hence improving general mental health.
- Improves digestion and relieves sleeplessness symptoms.

2. Seated Twist

Instructions:

1. Sit upright in a chair, feet flat on the floor.
2. Inhale to stretch your spine, then exhale and twist your torso to the right, with your left hand on your right knee and your right hand behind you on the chair.
3. Hold the twist for a few breaths, deepening with each exhalation.
4. Inhale to return to the center, then repeat on the left side.

Benefits:

❖ Enhances spinal mobility and flexibility.
❖ Massages the interior organs, promoting digestion.
❖ Helps to reduce tension in the back and shoulders.

3. Seated Leg Lifts

Instructions:

1. Sit up straight, back against the chair.
2. Extend your right leg straight in front of you, maintaining it parallel to the ground.
3. Hold for a few seconds, activating your core, before lowering it back down.
4. Repeat 10-15 times, then transfer to your left leg.

Benefits:

* ❖ Strengthens hip flexors and quads, improving muscle tone.
* ❖ Improves core stability and balance.
* ❖ Helps to burn calories and promotes weight loss.

4. Seated Cat-Cow

Instructions:

1. Sit upright with your feet flat on the floor and hands on your knees.
2. Inhale, arch your back and look upward (Cow Pose).
3. Exhale, round your back, and tuck your chin into your chest (Cat Pose).
4. Continue alternating between these two positions for 5-10 breaths.

Benefits:

* ❖ Improves spinal flexibility and posture.
* ❖ Releases stress in the back and neck.
* ❖ Promotes relaxation and stress reduction.

5. Seated Warrior 2

Instructions:

1. Sit tall in your chair, feet flat on the floor.
2. Extend your right leg to the side while keeping it straight, then bend your left knee.
3. Raise your arms parallel to the floor and look at your right fingertips.
4. Hold for a few breaths before switching sides.

Benefits:

- ❖ Increases lower body strength and stability.
- ❖ Enhances concentration and mental focus.
- ❖ Opens the hips and chest, increasing general flexibility.

6. Seated Sun Salutation

Instructions:

1. Sit tall with hands at the heart center.
2. Inhale, extending your arms upwards and stretching your spine.
3. Exhale and fold into a forward bend.
4. Inhale, raise back to the starting position and repeat the sequence numerous times.

Benefits:

- ❖ Boosts energy levels in both the body and mind.
- ❖ Enhances general flexibility and circulation.
- ❖ Breathing helps to promote mindfulness and relaxation.

7. Seated Pigeon Pose

Instructions:

1. Sit tall in your chair with your right ankle on your left knee.
2. Inhale to stretch your spine, then exhale as you softly lean forward with your back straight.
3. Maintain the stance for a few breaths, feeling the stretch in your hip.
4. Switch sides and repeat.

Benefits:

- ❖ Opens the hips, reducing tension and discomfort.
- ❖ Improves lower-body flexibility.
- ❖ Lowers tension and anxiety.

8. Chair's Extended Side Angle

Instructions:

1. Sit on the edge of your chair, feet firmly on the ground.
2. Extend your right arm above and lean to the left to perform a side stretch.
3. Rest your left hand on your left knee for support.
4. Hold for a few breaths, experiencing the stretch in your side body.
5. Switch sides and repeat.

Benefits:

❖ Increases flexibility in the spine and side body.
❖ It strengthens the core and obliques.
❖ Improves balance and coordination.

CHAPTER 5: CHAIR EXERCISES FOR PHYSICAL STRENGTH

1. Seated Banded Chest Press

Instructions:

1. Sit erect in a firm chair, feet level on the ground, back straight.
2. Wrap a resistance band over your back and fasten it at the back of the chair.
3. Hold the band handles at shoulder height, palms facing front, elbows bent 90 degrees.
4. Exhale and drive the grips forward, fully extending your arms with your elbows slightly bent.
5. Pause at the finish of the movement, then inhale and return to the beginning position with control.

Benefits:

❖ Improves upper body strength by strengthening pectoral, deltoids, and tricep muscles.
❖ Enhances shoulder stability and functional mobility.
❖ Can improve posture by strengthening the chest and shoulder muscles.

2. Seated Bicep Curls

Instructions:

1. Sit on a chair with a dumbbell in each hand, arms at your sides, palms forward.
2. Exhale as you curl the weights up towards your shoulders, keeping your elbows tight to your torso.
3. Squeeze your biceps at the apex of the movement, then inhale as you drop the weights back to their starting position.

Benefits:

* Isolates and strengthens the biceps, increasing arm strength and tone.
* Improves grip strength, which is essential for everyday activities.
* Facilitates functional movements, making tasks such as lifting objects easier.

3. Seated Shoulder Press

Instructions:

1. Sit on an upright chair with a dumbbell in each hand at shoulder height, palms facing forward.
2. Exhale while pressing the dumbbells overhead until your arms are fully stretched.

3. Lower the weights to shoulder height while breathing, keeping control throughout the exercise.

Benefits:

❖ Strengthens shoulder muscles for better overhead mobility and strength.
❖ Improves shoulder joint stability and reduces the chance of injury.
❖ Promotes good posture and upper-body strength.

4. Seated Eagle Pose

Instructions:

1. Sit up straight in a chair, feet flat on the ground.
2. Extend your arms in front of you, crossing one under the other.
3. Bend your elbows and bring your hands together, keeping this position for a few breaths.
4. Release and repeat on the opposite side.

Benefits:

❖ Increases upper body flexibility and range of motion in the shoulders.
❖ Relaxes and decreases tension in the upper back.

❖ Improves focus and concentration through mindful movement.

5. Seated Mountain Pose

Instructions:

1. Sit tall in a chair, feet flat on the floor, hands resting on knees.
2. Take a deep inhale, extending your arms aloft with your palms facing each other.
3. Maintain the pose for a few breaths, feeling the stretch in your spine.
4. Exhale and lower your arms to your knees.

Benefits:

❖ Improves core strength and postural stability.
❖ Improves awareness of breathing and body alignment.
❖ Focused breathing and stretching can help to reduce anxiety.

6. Seated Side Stretch

Instructions:

1. Sit tall in a chair, feet flat on the floor.
2. Raise your right arm overhead and bend to the left until you feel a stretch on your right side.

3. Hold for a few breaths before returning to the center and repeating on the opposite side.

Benefits:

* Increases spinal and torso flexibility.
* Helps to alleviate tension in the sides and lower back.
* Improves breathing patterns by expanding the chest and ribcage.

7. Modified Chair Squats

Instructions:

1. Sit on the edge of a sturdy chair, feet hip-width apart and flat on the floor.
2. Lean slightly forward and rise from your chair, using your core and leg muscles.
3. Carefully lower yourself back into the chair.

Benefits:

* Improves lower body strength, particularly the quadriceps, hamstrings, and glutes.
* Increases functional mobility, making it simpler to stand from a seated posture.
* Promotes equilibrium and stability.

8. Seated Toe Taps

Instructions:

1. Sit on a chair with feet flat on the floor.
2. Lift your right foot and tap your toes against the floor in front of you before returning to the beginning position.
3. Repeat with your left foot, alternating sides.

Benefits:

❖ Strengthens lower legs and increases ankle flexibility.
❖ Improves coordination and balance with controlled motions.
❖ Strengthens the muscles in the lower legs, which are necessary for daily tasks like as walking.

CHAPTER 6: CHAIR EXERCISES TO IMPROVE POSTURE

---

1. Seated Camel Pose

Instructions:

1. Sit tall on the edge of a sturdy chair, feet level on the floor, shoulder-width apart.
2. Inhale deeply, raising your chest and moving your shoulders back.
3. Exhale as you softly arch your back and reach your hands for your heels or the chair behind you.
4. Keep your neck flexible and avoid extending your head too far back.
5. Hold for 15-30 seconds while inhaling deeply.

Benefits:

* Stretches the front body and improving spinal flexibility.
* Strengthens back muscles, improving posture.
* Increases lung capacity and improves respiratory function.

2. Seated Happy Baby Pose

Instructions:

1. Sit on the edge of a chair, feet flat on the floor.
2. Bend your knees and lift your feet off the ground while holding your knees with your hands.
3. Pull your knees gently toward your armpits, maintaining your back straight.
4. Hold the position for 15-30 seconds while inhaling deeply.

Benefits:

❖ Reduces lower back strain and improves hip mobility.
❖ Improves flexibility in the groin and hip areas.
❖ Encourages relaxation and decreases tension.

3. Extended Triangle Pose

1. Sit with legs wide apart and feet flexed.
2. Inhale, raise your arms aloft and exhale as you bend toward one leg, hand on thigh, or foot.
3. Extend the other arm straight up while keeping your torso open.
4. Hold for 15-30 seconds and then switch sides.

Benefits:

❖ Enhances balance and coordination.
❖ Strengthens the legs while stretching the sides of the body.
❖ Increases flexibility and minimizes spinal tension.

4. Seated Half Lord of the Fishes

1. Sit tall on your chair, feet flat on the floor.
2. Place one hand behind you, and the other hand on the outside of the opposing knee.
3. Inhale to stretch your spine, then exhale as you gradually twist toward the back of the chair.
4. Hold for 15-30 seconds and then switch sides.

Benefits:

❖ Enhances spinal mobility and flexibility.
❖ Massages interior organs to improve digestion.
❖ Reduces stiffness in the back and shoulders.

5. Chair Spinal Twist

Instructions:

1. Sit upright in the chair, feet flat on the ground.
2. Inhale to stretch your spine, then exhale and twist your torso to one side, utilizing the backrest for support.

3. Hold for 15-30 seconds and then switch sides.

Benefits:

* ❖ Improves spinal flexibility and mobility.
* ❖ Reduces lower back discomfort by promoting proper alignment.
* ❖ Gentle belly massage helps to improve digestion.

6. Seated Reverse Warrior

Instructions:

1. Sit on the edge of a chair with legs extended wide.
2. Inhale and extend one arm overhead, leaning toward the opposing leg.
3. Hold the stance for 15-30 seconds, with your body extended and your neck relaxed.
4. Switch sides and repeat.

Benefits:

* ❖ Improves leg strength and side body flexibility.
* ❖ Enhances general balance and coordination.
* ❖ Increases lung capacity with deep, mindful breathing.

7. Seated Chest Opener

Instructions:

1. Sit at the edge of the chair, feet flat on the ground.
2. Inhale as you raise your arms to the sides, then clasp your hands behind your back.
3. Exhale and gently draw your shoulder blades together, elevating your chest.
4. Hold for 15-30 seconds while inhaling deeply.

Benefits:

❖ Opens the chest and improves posture.
❖ Releases tension in the shoulders and upper back.
❖ Improves breathing by extending the chest region.

8. Seated High Alternate Lean

Instructions:

1. Sit on the chair's edge with your feet on the floor.
2. Inhale, stretching both arms aloft, and exhale while leaning slightly to one side.
3. Hold for 15–30 seconds before returning to the center and switching sides.

Benefits:

- ❖ Improves lateral flexibility and stretches the sides of the torso.
- ❖ Promotes good posture by extending the spine.
- ❖ Increases blood flow throughout the body.

CHAPTER 7: CHAIR EXERCISES FOR FLEXIBILITY, MOBILITY, AND BALANCE

1. King Arthur's Pose

Instructions:

1. Sit tall in your chair, feet flat on the ground.
2. Extend one leg straight out in front, with the heel on the floor.
3. Slowly tilt forward from the hips, reaching for your extended foot with a flat back.
4. Hold the stretch for 20-30 seconds and then swap sides.

Benefits:

* Improves hamstring flexibility.
* Strengthens the lower back.
* Improves posture and relieves muscle tension in the legs.

2. Seated Tree Pose

Instructions:

1. Sit erect on your chair, feet flat on the floor.
2. Lift your right foot and rest the sole against the inner left thigh or calf.
3. Raise your arms upward, palms together.
4. Hold for 20-30 seconds and then switch legs.

Benefits:

* Enhances balance and coordination.
* It strengthens the core and leg muscles.
* Improves focus and bodily awareness.

3. Seated Bound Angle Pose

Instructions:

1. Sit at the edge of the chair, back straight.
2. Bring the soles of your feet together and slowly lower your knees to the sides.
3. Hold your feet with your hands while maintaining a long spine.
4. Hold the stance for 30 seconds to a minute.

Benefits:

* ❖ Stretches the hips, inner thighs, and groin.
* ❖ Improves hip flexibility.
* ❖ Improves the circulation in the lower body.

4. Extended Side Angle Pose

Instructions:

1. Sit erect with feet wide apart and toes pointed forward.
2. Raise your right arm toward the ceiling and rest your left elbow on your left thigh.
3. Stretch to the side while maintaining your chest open.
4. Hold for 20-30 seconds and then switch sides.

Benefits:

* ❖ Strengthens obliques and legs.
* ❖ Increases hip and spinal flexibility.
* ❖ Improves balance and stability.

5. Seated Sage 3 Pose

Instructions:

1. Sit tall on your chair and extend one leg straight in front.
2. Maintain a long spine by reaching your hands toward the foot of your outstretched leg.
3. Hold for 30 seconds and then switch sides.

Benefits:

❖ Increases hamstring and lower back length.
❖ Increases spinal flexibility.
❖ Improves posture and relieves stiffness.

6. Seated Wide-legged Forward Fold

Instructions:

1. Sit at the edge of the chair, feet apart.
2. Inhale to stretch your spine, then exhale and bend forward from your hips.
3. Rest your hands on the floor or your thighs while keeping your back flat.
4. Hold for 30 to 60 seconds.

Benefits:

* ❖ Stretches inner thighs and lower back.
* ❖ Improves hip mobility.
* ❖ Promotes relaxation by reducing tension in the lower body.

7. Seated Knee-to-Chest Pose

Instructions:

1. Sit tall in your chair, feet flat on the ground.
2. Bring one knee to your chest and hold it with both hands.
3. Gently move your knee closer while keeping your back straight.
4. Hold for 20-30 seconds and then switch legs.

Benefits:

* ❖ Stretches the lower back and hip flexors.
* ❖ Improves hip mobility.
* ❖ Releases stress in the lower spine.

8. Seated Tummy Twists

Instructions:

1. Sit erect, feet flat on the floor.
2. Twist your torso to the right while holding onto the side of the chair with your hands.
3. Hold your spine straight as you deepen the twist with each exhalation.
4. Hold for 20-30 seconds and then switch sides.

Benefits:

- ❖ Improves spinal flexibility.
- ❖ Improves digestion and decreases bloating.
- ❖ Strengthens core muscles.

CHAPTER 8: CHAIR EXERCISES FOR HEART HEALTH

---

1. Seated Forward Bent

Instructions:

1. Sit erect on a chair and place your feet flat on the floor.
2. Inhale, then raise your arms upwards.
3. Exhale as you lean forward at the hips, lowering your hands to the floor or resting them on your legs.
4. Hold for a few breaths, allowing your back to extend and your head to dangle low.
5. Inhale to get back to an upright position.

Benefits:

❖ Increases flexibility in the spine and hamstrings.
❖ Improves blood circulation throughout the body.
❖ Reduces stress and encourages relaxation.

2. Foot-to-seat Pose

Instructions:

1. Sit in a firm chair with a straight back and level feet.
2. Lift your right foot and rest it on your left thigh.
3. Hold your back straight and softly press down on your right knee to deepen the stretch.
4. Hold for a few breaths and then swap legs.

Benefits:

❖ Improves hip and thigh flexibility.
❖ Increases blood flow to the legs, which might assist to reduce stiffness.
❖ Improves posture by opening up the hips.

3. Palm Tree Pose

Instructions:

1. Sit tall in a chair, feet flat on the floor.
2. Inhale and raise your arms upwards, interlocking your fingers.
3. Reach up to the ceiling, lengthening your spine.
4. Hold for a few breaths and then drop your arms.

Benefits:

* Improves upper-body strength and flexibility.
* Promotes deep breathing, which improves heart health.
* Increases focus and balance, resulting in greater stability.

4. Triangle Pose

1. Sit in a chair with your right leg extended to the side and your foot flat on the floor.
2. Raise your left arm straight up and reach across your right leg to feel a stretch on your side.
3. Hold for a few breaths and then switch sides.

Benefits:

* Enhances side-body flexibility and core strength.
* Increases flexibility in the legs and hips, improving mobility.
* Encourages deep breathing, which may reduce blood pressure.

5. Seated Leg Stretches

Instructions:

1. Sit at the edge of your chair, feet flat on the floor.
2. Extend your right leg straight ahead of you, flexing your foot.
3. Hold for a few seconds to feel the stretch in your calf and hamstring.
4. Lower your leg and then swap to your left leg.

Benefits:

* Boosts flexibility in hamstrings and calves.
* Increases circulation in the legs, which benefits heart health.
* Helps to relieve muscle tightness.

6. Calf Stretches

Instructions:

1. Sit with your back straight and feet flat on the ground.
2. Extend one leg forward, heel on the floor, toes pointing up.
3. Lean slightly forward to feel the stretch in your calf.
4. Hold for a few breaths and then swap legs.

Benefits:

* ❖ Improves calves' flexibility and mobility.
* ❖ Promotes circulation, which is necessary for heart health.
* ❖ It helps to reduce cramps and stiffness in the lower legs.

7. Chair Squat

Instructions:

1. Sit at the edge of the chair, feet hip-width apart.
2. Lean forward slightly and rise off the chair with your legs, keeping your back straight.
3. To sit without using your hands, carefully lower back down.
4. Repeat a few times.

Benefits:

* ❖ Increases leg strength and balance.
* ❖ Improves heart health by increasing physical activity.
* ❖ Promotes greater coordination and steadiness.

8. Seated Knee to Chest Pose

Instructions:

1. Sit erect on your chair, feet level on the ground.
2. Bring one knee up to your chest and hold it with both hands.
3. Hold for a few breaths before lowering it back down and switching legs.

Benefits:

❖ Relieves stiffness in the lower back and hips.
❖ Improves circulation in the lower body.
❖ Encourages relaxation and decreases tension.

CHAPTER 9: CHAIR EXERCISES FOR WHEEL CHAIR USERS

1. Seated Chest Expansions

Instructions:

1. Sit upright in your wheelchair, back straight.
2. Hold a resistance band or keep your arms extended in front of you, shoulder height.
3. Slowly pull your arms outwards, stretching the band or spreading your arms to the sides with your elbows slightly bent.
4. Squeeze your shoulder blades together while expanding your chest.
5. Hold the position for a few seconds before returning to the beginning position.
6. Repeat 10-15 times.

Benefits:

❖ Enhances upper body strength and flexibility.
❖ Improves posture and spinal alignment by activating the upper back and chest muscles.
❖ Improves lung capacity and breathing efficiency.

2. Seated Side Arm Stretches

Instructions:

1. Sit upright in your wheelchair with your feet flat on the floor or footrests.
2. Raise one arm overhead and stretch to the opposing side.
3. Hold the stretch for 15-30 seconds while feeling the stretch down your side.
4. Return to the start position and repeat on the opposite side.
5. Repeat 5-10 times, alternating sides.

Benefits:

* Improves lateral flexibility and mobility in the torso.
* Helps to reduce tension in the shoulders and neck.
* Encourages deep breathing to promote relaxation and mental clarity.

3. Seated Dive Stretches

Instructions:

1. Sit upright in your wheelchair, feet flat on the floor.
2. Lean forward and extend your arms overhead, attempting to reach your toes or as far as you feel comfortable.
3. Maintain the position for a few seconds while breathing deeply.

4. Gradually return to an upright position.
5. Repeat 5-10 times.

Benefits:

* ❖ Stretches the lower back, hamstrings, and shoulders.
* ❖ Enhances general flexibility and range of motion.
* ❖ Controls movement, promotes relaxation and stress relief.

4. Seated Raised Arm Circles

Instructions:

1. Sit upright in your wheelchair, feet flat on the ground.
2. Extend your arms to the sides, shoulder height.
3. Begin by drawing little circles with your arms, gradually increasing the size of the circles.
4. Make 10 circles in one direction, then switch to the other direction.
5. Ensure that your core is engaged during the action.

Benefits:

* ❖ Improves shoulder mobility and stability.
* ❖ Improves circulation to the arms and upper body.
* ❖ Helps to reduce stiffness and stress in the shoulder joints.

5. Seated Overhead Punches

Instructions:

1. Sit erect with feet firmly on the ground.
2. Raise your right arm overhead, as if punching upward.
3. Return to the beginning position, then repeat with the left arm.
4. Repeat 10-15 times per arm, alternating between them.

Benefits:

* Strengthens shoulders, arms, and upper chest.
* Improves coordination and rhythm.
* Improves cardiovascular health by increasing heart rate during exercise.

6. Seated Hip Stretches

Instructions:

1. Sit upright in your wheelchair with your back straight.
2. Put one ankle on the other knee.
3. Gently press down on the lifted knee to increase the stretch.
4. Hold the stretch for 15–30 seconds before switching legs.
5. Repeat 5-10 stretches for each side.

Benefits:

❖ Improves hip flexibility.
❖ It relieves stress and soreness in the lower body.
❖ Improves blood flow to the lower extremities.

7. Seated Leg Stretches

Instructions:

1. Sit erect, back straight, and feet level on the floor.
2. Extend one leg straight in front of you, maintaining it parallel with the ground.
3. Hold the position for a few seconds before lowering your leg back down.
4. Repeat for the opposite leg.
5. Do 5-10 reps per leg.

Benefits:

❖ Enhances leg strength and mobility.
❖ Stretches the hamstrings and calves.
❖ Improves lower-body coordination and stability.

8. Seated Twist

Instructions:

1. Sit upright in your wheelchair, feet flat.
2. With your right hand on the back of the wheelchair, swivel your torso to the right.
3. Hold the position for 15-30 seconds while feeling the stretch in your back.
4. Return to the center, then repeat on the left side.
5. Repeat 5-10 times, alternating sides.

Benefits:

❖ Improves spine flexibility and mobility.
❖ Releases stress in the back and shoulders.
❖ Improves core stability and strength.

CHAPTER 10: STAYING MOTIVATED AND OVERCOMING CHALLENGES

Common Obstacles To Exercise And How To Address Them

Exercise provides several physical, mental, and emotional benefits, especially for seniors who want to maintain or enhance their health. Despite the documented benefits, many older persons face major impediments to regular physical activity. Recognizing and conquering these challenges is critical for remaining active and living a healthier, more independent lifestyle. Below, we look at some typical hurdles to fitness for seniors and offer practical solutions to overcome them.

1. Physical Limitations

As people age, they frequently develop physical restrictions such as joint discomfort, arthritis, or diminished mobility. These difficulties might make traditional types of exercise appear intimidating, causing fear of damage or discomfort. For seniors who are already managing chronic diseases, the prospect of beginning an exercise routine may be overwhelming.

How to Overcome Physical Limitations

❖ **Begin with Low-Impact Exercises:** Seniors can benefit from low-impact activities including chair exercises, swimming, and walking. These exercises put less load on the joints while increasing strength and flexibility. Chair exercises, for example, allow people to focus on multiple muscle groups while remaining sitting, lowering their risk of injury.

❖ **Modify workouts to Fit Your Ability:** Many workouts can be tailored to certain physical constraints. Exercises such as squats or lunges, for example, can be performed with a chair for support, lessening the intensity but maintaining the benefits. Gentle range-of-motion exercises can help relieve stiffness and improve movement in severe arthritis patients.

❖ **Consult with a Healthcare Professional:** Before starting any new fitness plan, seniors should consult with their healthcare professional or physical therapist to see which exercises are appropriate for their medical circumstances.

2. Fear of Injuries or Falls

Fear of injury, particularly falls, is a prominent concern among older persons. Individuals who are afraid of falling may avoid activities that involve balance or coordination, such as walking on uneven surfaces, standing exercises, or weight-bearing actions. This dread frequently leads to inactivity, which can harm physical health and increase the risk of falls caused by weakening muscles.

How to Handle Fear of Injury:

❖ **Focus on Balance and Strength Training:** Including balance and strength exercises in your training routine will greatly lower the danger of falling. Chair exercises are very beneficial for seniors who are concerned about balance. Exercises such as seated marches and seated leg lifts serve to strengthen the legs and core, which improves stability.

❖ **Use Support Assistance:** When exercising, seniors can use assistance such as chairs, handrails, or even resistance bands to help them maintain balance and avoid falls. For example, a chair can be utilized to offer stability to standing workouts.

❖ **Build Confidence Gradually:** It's critical to begin slowly and gradually increase your confidence. Begin with simple, low-intensity exercises and progressively increase the challenge as your strength and balance improve. This incremental method allows seniors to feel more safe and less afraid of damage as they improve their skills.

3. Lack of Motivation

Many people struggle to remain motivated to exercise. Seniors may be unmotivated because of past failures, a lack of immediate results, or feelings of exhaustion. Without a planned plan or external support, it is simple to become inactive.

How to Deal with Lack of Motivation:

❖ Having small, realistic goals is essential for staying motivated. Goals like "walking for 10 minutes a day" or "performing three chair exercises each week" are attainable and contribute to a sense of success. As progress is accomplished, these objectives might be altered to keep the sense of challenge and growth.

❖ Consistency is essential for remaining motivated. A regular exercise program, such as setting out specified days and times for exercise, can assist seniors in incorporating exercise into their daily lives. This decreases the mental work required to begin a session, making it simpler to sustain momentum.

❖ Exercising with a friend, or family member, or in a group environment can enhance the experience and promote accountability. Social involvement is a powerful motivator, and sharing your workout adventure with others might help you stick to a fitness plan. Many towns have senior-friendly exercise courses, either in person or online, that combine health and social interaction.

4. Limited Access to Exercise Facilities and Equipment

Not everyone has access to gyms, pools, or specialized fitness equipment. This lack of availability can deter seniors from starting or sustaining a fitness regimen, especially if they believe they require certain equipment to exercise.

How to Handle Limited Access:

- ❖ **Exercise at Home:** Many excellent workouts can be performed in the comfort of one's own home using little or no equipment. Chair workouts, bodyweight exercises, and stretching routines are all good examples of activities that require little room and equipment. A solid chair and resistance bands are frequent enough to execute a wide range of strengthening and mobility exercises.

- ❖ **Use Online Resources:** There are numerous online platforms that provide free or low-cost workout regimens geared toward elders. These can be accessible from a computer, tablet, or smartphone, allowing seniors to complete supervised workouts at home. Look for programs designed expressly for older individuals, with modifications to accommodate varying abilities.

❖ **Explore Community Resources:** Many local community centers, senior centers, and recreation facilities provide low-cost or free exercise programs for seniors. These programs frequently involve group courses, swimming, or walking groups, which give a structured setting for staying active.

5. Fatigue and Lack of Energy

Fatigue is a prevalent problem among seniors, especially those who have chronic illnesses like heart disease or diabetes. This lack of energy might make the prospect of exercising appear laborious or overwhelming. However, consistent physical activity has been demonstrated to enhance energy levels over time, making it an essential component of fatigue management.

How to Treat Fatigue:

❖ **Start Slowly and Listen to Your Body:** For seniors coping with weariness, it's critical to begin with short, reasonable activity sessions. Begin with just 5-10 minutes of light movement, such as sitting exercises or slow-paced walking, and gradually increase as your energy levels improve.

❖ **Incorporate recovery Days:** While consistency is key, it is also critical to allow for enough recovery between training sessions. Rest days allow the body to recoup and recharge, which helps elders manage fatigue while remaining active.

❖ **Exercise at Your Best Time:** Some people feel more energized at specific times of the day. Seniors should exercise when they have the most energy, whether it is in the morning, afternoon, or evening. This might make the workout less tiring and more pleasurable.

6. Chronic Health Conditions

Chronic health disorders such as diabetes, heart disease, or pulmonary issues can make exercise appear difficult or dangerous. Seniors may be unaware of what sorts of physical activity are safe for their condition, leading to a lack of exercise altogether.

How to Treat Chronic Health Conditions:

❖ **Work with a Healthcare Provider:** Before beginning any exercise program, it is critical to check with a doctor, particularly for seniors with chronic diseases. A healthcare expert can propose specific activities that are both safe and useful, taking into account any limits or threats to the individual's health.

❖ **Focus on Gentle, Consistent Activity:** Even for elders with chronic diseases, frequent physical activity is essential for symptom management and overall health. Low-intensity workouts such as chair yoga, strolling, or stretching can assist improve cardiovascular health, strength, and flexibility without putting undue stress on the body.

Addressing these frequent barriers can help seniors incorporate regular exercise into their lives, thereby increasing their health, mobility, and quality of life. Overcoming these challenges, whether through changes, social support, or individualized routines, can lead to a more active and meaningful existence.

Tips For Maintaining Motivation And Accountability

Staying motivated and accountable in a fitness plan can be difficult at times, especially for seniors who participate in chair exercises. Life's challenges, health difficulties, or simply a lack of energy can all make it difficult to stay active. However, with the correct mindset and tactics, remaining on track with your fitness objectives is both attainable and satisfying. Let's look at some practical ways to assist elders in staying motivated and accountable as they work toward greater health using chair exercises.

1. Set Clear and Realistic Goals

Setting specific and attainable goals is one of the most efficient methods to maintain motivation. Setting clear goals for your fitness journey provides you with a sense of direction and purpose. These objectives should be attainable and suited to your fitness level. For example, if you're just getting started with chair exercises, set a goal of 15 minutes of activity three times each week. As you progress, progressively increase the duration or intensity.

It is critical to avoid establishing overly ambitious goals, which may lead to dissatisfaction or harm. Break down huge ambitions into smaller, more doable benchmarks. Every time you reach one of these milestones, you feel a sense of success and inspiration to keep going.

2. Track Your Progress

Tracking your success is vital for keeping you accountable. When you can see the effects of your efforts, you feel a sense of accomplishment and are motivated to keep going. Keeping a fitness journal is an excellent way to record your workouts, recording the exercises you did, how you felt during the session, and any gains in strength, flexibility, or endurance.

Additionally, some elders find digital fitness trackers useful. These devices can track your activity, calories expended, and even heart rate during exercise. Whether you use a traditional notebook or a technological technique, documenting your development can keep you aware of your progress, which can be a powerful motivation.

3. Create a Routine

Establishing a consistent fitness program is critical to developing long-term habits. Routine reduces the need to make daily decisions about whether or not to exercise because it is already planned into your schedule. It's a good idea to schedule your chair workouts on set days and times and stick to them like any other appointment.

For example, on Mondays, Wednesdays, and Fridays, you could arrange your workouts immediately after breakfast. A schedule can add a feeling of normalcy and structure to your week, making it easier to stick to even on days when motivation is low. Over time, consistency will allow your workout regimen to become a normal part of your daily life.

4. Make it fun

Exercise does not have to feel like a hassle. One approach to keep motivated is to make your chair workout regimen fun. You can accomplish this by combining activities that you enjoy or making minor adjustments to keep things exciting. For example, when exercising, listen to your favorite music or audiobook. Music has a profound effect on mood and energy levels, making you feel more involved and excited about your workout.

You might also try exercising in a new setting. If feasible, perform your chair exercises outside on a sunny day. Fresh air and a change of environment can help you stay motivated and appreciate the experience more. Finding methods to include pleasure and excitement into your workout regimen might make all the difference in keeping motivated in the long run.

5. Seek Support from Family and Friends

Staying accountable can be made much easier with the help of others. Involving family members, friends, or even a workout buddy can help you stay motivated and encouraged on days when you don't feel like exercising. You may invite a friend or family member to participate in your chair exercises, either in person or digitally via a video call. Exercising with others may transform your workout into a social affair, making it more pleasurable and less like a single effort.

Sharing your health objectives with a loved one might also help you stay accountable. They can check in with you regularly to see how your workouts are going and provide positive feedback. Knowing that someone else is pulling for your success can provide the extra motivation you need to be consistent.

6. Reward Yourself

Rewarding oneself for achieving goals or completing workouts is another effective approach to staying motivated. These rewards do not have to be pricey; they can be as basic as eating your favorite snack or devoting time to a hobby you enjoy. The idea is to connect your accomplishments to happy experiences.

For example, after a week of consistent chair exercises, reward yourself with a soothing bath or an episode of your favorite TV show. These small incentives can start a positive feedback loop, strengthening your dedication to your fitness regimen. Celebrating your achievement, no matter how tiny, can help you stay enthusiastic and motivated.

7. Focus on the Benefits

It's easy to lose sight of why you started exercising in the first place, especially on days when you're not feeling particularly energetic or inspired. To combat this, remind yourself on a regular basis of the benefits of chair exercises. Whether it's increasing your mobility, flexibility, or mental wellness, concentrating on the good outcomes can rekindle your enthusiasm.

Keep a list of your reasons for exercising somewhere visible, such as on your refrigerator or bathroom mirror. This visual reminder will serve as a daily nudge, keeping you focused on your "why" and maintaining a good attitude toward your fitness path.

8. Adapt to Challenges

Maintaining an exercise program might be difficult at times due to life's demands. Challenges are unavoidable, whether they are related to health, a hectic schedule, or a lack of energy. Learning to adapt is essential for keeping motivated and accountable. If you skip a day or two of exercise, don't be too hard on yourself; simply start up where you left off.

Flexibility is essential, particularly as you traverse the ups and downs of life. If you aren't feeling up to your typical program, you can change the exercises or do a shorter session. The key thing is to keep moving, even if at a slower rate. Being adaptive allows you to overcome temporary setbacks while maintaining your pace.

9. Join a Senior Fitness Group

Joining a senior exercise club or class, whether in person or online, can help you remain on track while also offering a sense of community. Many seniors find that being part of a group helps them stay motivated and involved. Group settings allow for social connection, support, and a shared sense of purpose. When you know that others are joining you, it is easier to show up and put in the effort.

Online platforms now provide a wide range of fitness sessions specifically designed for elders, including chair exercise routines. These classes provide discipline and advice, allowing you to stay on track while connecting with people who have similar fitness goals.

10. Visualize Your Success

Visualization is a crucial tool for staying motivated. Spend a few minutes each day seeing yourself succeeding in your fitness path, whether that means decreasing weight, feeling stronger, or regaining mobility. Visualizing your future self-reaping the benefits of regular exercise helps motivate you to keep going, even if progress seems slow.

By focusing on the positive results you want to achieve, you develop a mental image that strengthens your resolve. This optimistic vision might help you stay motivated by making your long-term goals feel more tangible and achievable.

Staying motivated and accountable in any fitness regimen is critical, especially for a senior looking to enhance their health through chair exercises. With the appropriate tactics in place, you can overcome challenges, maintain consistency, and reach your fitness objectives while enjoying the ride.

Celebrating Achievements

Celebrating accomplishments, no matter how minor, is an effective approach to keep motivated in your fitness path. Whether you're doing chair exercises to improve mobility, lose weight, or reclaim independence, marking milestones keeps your thinking positive and reinforces the behaviors that contribute to long-term success.

Celebrating your fitness accomplishments extends beyond the physical advantages. It is crucial to maintain the mental and emotional motivation required for long-term success. *Here's why recognizing milestones is important:*

1. **Increases Motivation:** Motivation might diminish when results take time to materialize, particularly in fitness. Celebrating even modest victories, such as finishing a week of chair exercises or improving posture, reinforces your success and keeps you motivated to keep going.

2. **Increases Confidence:** Many seniors start their fitness journey with reservations about their skills, especially if they haven't worked out in years or are recovering from an ailment. Celebrating each step forward tells you that you are capable of developing and improving. Confidence grows when you see yourself mastering new activities or achieving personal goals.

3. **Reinforces Positive Behavior:** Recognizing your accomplishments allows you to reward yourself for your hard work. This establishes a positive feedback loop in which your brain equates hard labor with happy emotions, making you more likely to adhere to your habit.

4. **Improves Mental Health:** Exercise naturally boosts mood by producing endorphins, but celebrating accomplishments adds an extra layer of happiness. Recognizing your success improves your mental well-being and reduces frustration, which can emerge when you don't notice immediate effects.

5. **Prevents Burnout:** Many people become disheartened when their goals seem far away or the path ahead appears long. Breaking down your fitness journey into smaller, more manageable steps will help you avoid burnout. Celebrating each step reminds you that you are making progress, which helps you avoid feeling overwhelmed.

Practical Ways to Celebrate Achievements

Once you've identified your accomplishments, the following step is to celebrate. *Here are some healthy and meaningful ways of acknowledging your accomplishments:*

1. **Set mini-goals and reward yourself:** Break down your major fitness goals into smaller, more doable benchmarks.

For example, if you aim to complete a 30-day chair exercise challenge, give yourself a modest reward at the end of each week, such as a favorite healthy treat, a new book, or a day off.

2. **Start a Progress Journal:** Keep a journal in which you record your daily or weekly accomplishments. Write down how you felt after doing your workouts, make any improvements, and reflect on your achievements. Looking back through your notebook can provide a significant boost of motivation when you need it the most.

3. **Celebrate with Others:** Sharing your accomplishments with friends, family, or a fitness club may be quite fulfilling. Not only does this build a supportive group around you, but it also helps you stay focused on your goals. You may even encourage others to begin their fitness adventures.

4. **Take Progress Photos or Videos:** Visualizing your progress may be extremely encouraging. Take images or videos of yourself performing specific workouts at various phases throughout your trip. When you notice changes in your posture, flexibility, or strength, you will be reminded of how far you have come.

5. **Treat Yourself to Fitness Gear:** As you complete key milestones, consider rewarding yourself with new fitness equipment. A new pair of shoes, resistance bands, or comfy

training clothing can make your workout regimen feel new and interesting.

6. **Plan a Special Outing:** Recognize your accomplishments by engaging in a fun, healthful activity you enjoy. This could include a nature walk, a day at the park with family, or a soothing spa day. Doing something that makes you happy is an excellent approach to reinforcing the positive feelings linked with your hard work.

7. **Reflect on the Bigger Picture:** Sometimes the best way to celebrate is to simply take a moment to consider the big picture. Recognize your physical, mental, and emotional progress, and give yourself credit for taking control of your health. Remember that the fitness journey is ongoing, and each step forward is worth celebrating.

Celebrating milestones not only makes your fitness journey more pleasurable but also helps to ensure long-term success. When you reward yourself for your efforts and achievements, you're more likely to stick to your goals. This establishes a continuous cycle of drive, growth, and fulfillment.

Celebrating your milestones, no matter how large or small, gives you the motivation you need to keep going, no matter what obstacles you face.

Inspirational Stories Of Elders Who Benefited From Chair Exercises

As we age, the physical obstacles we confront might become daunting. Staying active might be challenging for seniors due to physical pain, diminished flexibility, and exhaustion. Chair exercises, on the other hand, have proven to be a simple and effective method of maintaining physical health and independence. These exercises are gentle but effective, making them ideal for seniors who may struggle with mobility but want to keep active. Here are a few inspiring anecdotes about seniors who have benefited from chair exercises, demonstrating how transformative they can be in enhancing quality of life.

Margaret, Chicago

Margaret, 75, has spent the majority of her life being physically active, going for long walks and attending community fitness courses. However, following hip surgery and a series of problems, she was largely restricted to her home, relying heavily on her walker. The loss of her independence was difficult to endure. She struggled to accomplish daily tasks like cooking and cleaning, and her lack of freedom resulted in a time of sadness and dissatisfaction.

Margaret opted to attempt chair exercises after her physical therapist suggested them. She started with easy seated exercises to regain leg strength and enhance her balance. Over time, the workouts helped her rebuild muscular tone and flexibility, particularly in her lower body, which had deteriorated following surgery.

What surprised Margaret the most was not only the physical benefits, but also how much her emotional health improved. The greater mobility offered her a renewed sense of hope and independence. Margaret now does her chair exercises daily and has started attending a local senior fitness club that incorporates similar moves. She is pleased to report that she no longer needs her walker at home and can now make meals for herself. Margaret's tale demonstrates the efficacy of chair exercises in restoring physical and emotional well-being.

John, Kansas City

At the age of 78, John was battling with weight gain, which had a severe impact on his mobility and overall health. He struggled to walk for long periods, and his sedentary lifestyle contributed to more weight difficulties. His doctor cautioned him that unless he made adjustments, he could develop significant health concerns such as heart disease and diabetes. John thought exercise was impossible because he suffered from joint pain and shortness of breath even when standing or walking short distances.

To help John get started on his fitness journey, a community senior center introduced him to chair exercises that focused on low-impact mobility. The seated workouts helped him to strengthen his legs, arms, and core without putting undue strain on his joints. As he gradually added more difficult activities, John's weight and energy levels began to shift.

John shed 30 pounds over a year. This weight loss was more than simply statistics; it also enhanced his mobility and confidence. He discovered that as he developed his muscles and improved his balance with chair exercises, simple actions such as getting out of a chair, mounting stairs, and even going for short walks were simpler. Now, John adds chair exercises into his daily routine, frequently guiding his fellow elders in group sessions. His tale demonstrates that it is never too late to lose weight and improve health, regardless of starting point.

Betty, Oakland

Betty, 82, struggled with persistent pain caused by arthritis regularly. Getting out of bed, sitting in a chair, and even carrying a cup of tea became unpleasant. Betty was always a gregarious person who enjoyed gardening and attending church events, but her discomfort had caused her to retreat from these activities. Her doctor had suggested a variety of treatments, but none appeared to provide long-term comfort.

Betty decided to attempt chair workouts after a friend suggested them to her. She was first doubtful about the potential benefits of such delicate movements, but she was prepared to give it a shot. Her instructor taught her stretches and motions that targeted specific areas of discomfort, such as her hips, knees, and lower back.

Betty felt less pain after a few weeks of consistent practice. The low-impact nature of the exercises allowed her to move without hurting her arthritis, while the moderate stretching helped alleviate joint stiffness. She was soon able to resume her regular activities without feeling as uncomfortable as before. Betty's chair exercises not only helped her physical health but also allowed her to return to activities she enjoyed, such as gardening and attending social events at her local church.

Frank, Berlin

Frank, 83, has a history of heart problems. Following a heart attack a few years ago, his doctor encouraged him to stay physically active to maintain his cardiovascular health. Frank, on the other hand, was wary of typical workout programs because he thought they were too intense and worried about overexertion.

A local fitness group suggested chair exercises as a method to preserve cardiovascular health without going overboard. Frank started with easy seated motions that engaged his core, arms, and legs while keeping his heart rate within a safe range. The modest aerobic activities, such as seated marches and toe taps, gradually improved his endurance.

Frank's endurance improved over time, as did his overall energy levels. More importantly, frequent chair workouts helped him maintain a healthy heart while reducing his risk of injury or overexertion. His doctor was impressed by the excellent impact these workouts had on Frank's heart health, and he now urges other seniors in his town to follow suit.

Evelyn, Maryland

Evelyn, 86, had always taken pride in her independence, but after a few falls, she began to fear getting around on her own. Her dread of falling again made her feel vulnerable, resulting in a dramatic decrease in her activity levels. She grew very reliant on others, which annoyed her greatly.

Chair exercises that emphasized balance and mobility provided Evelyn with the confidence she needed to regain control of her body. She felt more confident after doing movements that strengthened her core and improved her stability, such as seated leg lifts and torso twists. These exercises also enhanced her reaction time, allowing her to recover faster if she lost her balance.

Evelyn's balance improved dramatically after several months of practice with these exercises. She now moves boldly around her home and has reclaimed much of her freedom. Her experience demonstrates how chair exercises can help seniors avoid falls and provide the security and confidence they need to remain active and independent.

These anecdotes about seniors who have benefited from chair exercises show how beneficial these routines can be to their physical, emotional, and mental health. Whether it's regaining independence, losing weight, managing chronic pain, maintaining heart health, or improving balance, chair exercises make it easy for seniors to stay active and enjoy life to the fullest. These inspiring people demonstrate that it is never too late to enhance one's health and rediscover a sense of purpose through activity.

Encouragement For Readers To Share Their Journey

Sharing personal health and exercise experiences, particularly in later life, can be one of the most inspiring and influential things a senior can do. Seniors benefit not only directly from sharing their path, but also from inspiring others, making connections, and cultivating a sense of community around health and wellness. Whether it's sharing milestones, problems, or little successes, talking about one's fitness journey—especially when it comes to chair exercises—can result in a slew of emotional, mental, and social benefits.

1. Establishing a Sense of Community and Connection

One of the most important advantages of documenting your fitness journey is the sense of community it develops. Fitness and health are universal issues, particularly for seniors, and chair exercises are frequently something that many people in comparable situations can connect to. When you share your story, whether with family, friends or on social media, you open the door to connecting with others who may be on the same journey or seeking direction and support.

Sharing your fitness journey helps to foster a friendly environment in which others feel less alone in their problems or worries. In a world where many seniors may feel alone, particularly owing to reduced mobility, reaching out via personal experiences might motivate others to take the first steps toward better health. As you share the ups and downs of your journey, you'll most likely meet people who share your experiences, forming a community in which everyone feels inspired and empowered to keep going forward.

2. Motivating Others to Take Action

Many seniors may be cautious or unsure about beginning a fitness regimen, especially if they have been inactive for a long period or have physical restrictions. When you share your experience, whether through anecdotes, images, films, or simply casual conversations, you can serve as a light of hope for those who are scared to start.

Your tale of overcoming obstacles, beginning with easy chair exercises and gradually increasing strength, flexibility, and endurance, can inspire others that it's never too late to improve their health. Your accomplishments, no matter how minor they appear, are invaluable to someone who is just getting started. By sharing, you demonstrate that even limited mobility is not a barrier to enhancing one's physical and mental health. You become an example for others to follow, encouraging them to take the initial step, no matter how tiny it is.

It's important to remember that even if you don't consider yourself a fitness guru or professional, your own experience is really valuable. People are typically more motivated by stories from peers than by specialists because they recognize themselves in the experience of someone who is similar to them. Your honesty, openness, and progress have the potential to inspire others to change.

3. Celebrating Milestones, Large and Small

When you share your path, you provide a chance to celebrate your accomplishments with others. These milestones can include reducing weight, increasing flexibility, or simply being able to complete an exercise that was previously difficult. Celebrating these triumphs, no matter how big or small, reinforces your progress and motivates you to keep working toward your goals.

As you share your accomplishments, others will cheer you on, offering encouragement and support. This sensation of praise and approval can increase your incentive to stay on course. Furthermore, by publicly celebrating your accomplishments, you may feel more responsibility to keep pushing yourself, knowing that people are rooting for you.

Celebrating milestones is about more than simply your own development; it is about offering others hope and support. When people witness you achieving your goals, they will understand that they, too, can achieve something significant in their fitness path. Sharing tales about overcoming obstacles, whether it's dealing with physical restrictions, finding the desire to exercise on a regular basis, or learning new motions, exhibits tenacity and can motivate others to celebrate their own accomplishments along the journey.

4. Increasing Accountability and Motivation

Maintaining motivation and consistency is one of the most difficult aspects of any fitness program. Sharing your journey with a community or close group of friends fosters a sense of accountability. When others are aware of your goals and progress, you may feel more motivated to stay in your routine since you know they are following and supporting you.

This is not to say that sharing puts pressure on others; rather, it motivates them. For example, publishing updates on your chair exercises or fitness routine on social media can provide positive feedback from friends and family, encouraging you to keep going. Similarly, discussing your success in senior fitness clubs or local exercise classes can spark significant conversations that not only motivate you but also allow you to benefit from the experiences of others.

Sharing your story does not require you to focus just on the positives; being open about troubles, disappointments, and challenges is also beneficial. When you discuss the difficult days, when training feels like a chore, or when progress appears slow, you promote a realistic view of the fitness journey. And when you get encouragement from those who understand your hardships, it helps to reconfirm that obstacles are part of the journey. This candid back-and-forth can create new encouragement to persevere.

5. Promoting Emotional and Mental Growth

Sharing your journey is about more than just physical fitness; it's also about the emotional and mental growth that comes with adopting a healthy lifestyle. Chair exercises can be extremely beneficial to your mental health, reducing stress, anxiety, and even symptoms of depression. When you share these mental health benefits, you help people understand the entire range of advantages that regular exercise provides.

Many seniors believe that remaining active is essential for maintaining independence, confidence, and general enjoyment. Sharing tales about how chair exercises have improved your quality of life—whether through more energy, better mobility, or simply feeling more in control of your body—can motivate others to take action for their own mental health. Letting people realize that exercise is about more than just physical fitness, but also about emotional well-being, broadens the conversation and makes fitness more accessible to individuals who are afraid to begin.

6. Leaving a Legacy of Health

Finally, sharing your fitness experience allows you to make a lasting impression on others. Sharing your story with family, friends, or even a larger audience helps to build a legacy of health and well-being. Your path can motivate not only your contemporaries but also future generations, demonstrating that fitness and self-care are lifetime hobbies.

You may discover that sharing your story inspires others to get involved—whether it's a friend starting their own chair exercise regimen, a family member joining you in your workouts, or someone online reaching out to express how your story inspired them. In this approach, you're establishing a chain reaction that promotes healthy lifestyles throughout many communities.

Sharing your chair exercise experience not only helps you improve your own health but also shows others that they, too, can do it. Every tale, whether about modest successes or huge milestones, has the potential to inspire, motivate, and effect substantial change.

CONCLUSION

As we near the end of this masterpiece, it's vital to pause and reflect on everything you've learned and accomplished thus far. Chair exercises may appear easy, yet they can have a significant influence on your general health and well-being. By committing to these workouts, you've taken a huge step toward a healthier, more active, and self-sufficient lifestyle.

One of the most essential takeaways from this book is the value of consistency. Consistency is essential whether you want to reduce weight, gain physical strength, improve your posture, or increase your flexibility and mobility. Chair exercises, when done frequently, can help you maintain and even increase your physical abilities as you age. You've learned how to incorporate these exercises into your daily routine, making fitness a regular part of your life.

Exercise, particularly as we age, is about more than simply physical strength. It's also about retaining freedom, remaining mobile, and improving your general quality of life. You've already taken the first step by learning the exercises in this book; now the challenge is to keep practicing them. This will provide you with long-term benefits, including incremental gains in your strength, flexibility, balance, and overall fitness.

Many seniors find it difficult to maintain a healthy weight as they become older due to changes in metabolism and physical activity levels. The chair exercises in this book are a practical and safe technique to help you achieve your weight management goals. These workouts not only burn calories but also improve muscular tone, which can boost metabolism over time.

Losing weight is about improving your complete health, not just your appearance. Excess weight can put undue strain on your joints, raise your risk of heart disease, and cause mobility issues. By following the chair exercise routines suggested in the book, you've given yourself the tools to counteract these health concerns while also improving your overall well-being. Remember that every modest effort matters and every workout session helps to build a healthier physique.

Independence is one of the most important parts of life as we age. The capacity to move freely, complete daily duties with ease, and traverse the world on your own terms is something we frequently take for granted in our youth. However, as mobility declines, many elders become concerned about losing their independence.

The exercises in this book are intended to help you reclaim and maintain your sense of independence. Improving your strength, balance, and flexibility gives you the best opportunity to continue to live life on your own terms. Simple movements like getting out of a chair, reaching for goods, and going upstairs become easier as your muscles strengthen and coordinate. These chair exercises, while easy and low-impact, have the ability to significantly enhance your functional fitness, allowing you to continue doing what you enjoy without relying on others.

One of the greatest advantages of chair exercises is their adjustability. Whether you're new to fitness or have been exercising for years, chair workouts can be tailored to your current fitness level. This makes them a fantastic choice for seniors of all skill levels. Throughout the book, I've included variations and tweaks to guarantee that every one may take part, regardless of physical restrictions.

The exercises in this book are designed for wheelchair users or those with limited mobility. They focus on crucial areas such as upper body strength, flexibility, and cardiovascular health. These exercises are designed to deliver excellent workouts while seated so that everyone can benefit from a regular fitness regimen.

If you ever feel like particular workouts are too difficult, remember that it's okay to begin slowly and gradually increase the intensity over time. The goal is not perfection, but growth. Listen to your body, be aware of your limitations, and modify your workout plan accordingly. The beauty of chair workouts is that they may progress alongside you as your strength and mobility improve.

Every fitness journey presents its own set of hurdles. Whether it's finding time to exercise, coping with health difficulties, or staying motivated in the face of adversity, it's critical to acknowledge that hurdles are a natural part of the process. The trick is to keep moving forward, even when it's difficult.

Chair exercises promote a sense of community, which is one of its most inspirational aspects. Seniors all over the world have embraced chair exercises as a method to improve their health and interact with others who have similar aims. You are not alone on this path. Whether you attend local classes, or online groups, or simply share your success with friends and family, remember that you are part of a supportive network of individuals who are working toward the same goals.

As you finish this book, consider it a new beginning. The exercises and routines you've learned will serve you well throughout your life. The journey to better health, mobility, and independence does not end here; it is an ongoing process.

Through these chair exercises, you've created habits, strength, and confidence that will serve you well in the years ahead. Whether you want to maintain your current fitness level, enhance your mobility, or just stay active as you get older, the information in this book will give you the tools you need to take control of your health.

As you progress, keep this book handy as a reference whenever you need advice, inspiration, or motivation. Chair exercises are a long-term, efficient strategy to maintain fitness and health, regardless of age or fitness level. Your dedication to your well-being demonstrates your strength, resilience, and determination.

Thank you for taking on this trip. Now it's time to apply what you've learned and continue living the healthier, more independent life you deserve.